A Century
of
Naturopathy

C.P. Negri, OMD, NMD

A Century of Naturopathy

By C.P. Negri, OMD, NMD

First Edition
Copyright 2013 C.P. Negri

Printed in the United States of America.

ISBN: 978-0-9819884-6-7

PREFACE

Writing a thorough history of Naturopathy posed something of a problem for me. First of all, no one had ever written a comprehensive book such as this one before —with good reason, as I found out. It is hard work.

Some of the few available books, such as Kirchfeld and Boyle's excellent *Nature Doctors*, give good biographical profiles of major figures in the field. But they do not give the reader a picture of the "personality" of the profession itself, as it has developed from its infancy through adolescence and now to maturity. It was only possible to do that by making a chronicle of events in a year-by-year fashion. In this way the new reader first becomes familiar with what comprises this wonderful approach to health care, then follows it as it picks up momentum and finally emerges after a century in the form that exists today.

And therein lies the other problem in writing this book. In depicting its rise and fall, and rise again, it is impossible to accurately portray the naturopathic field without exposing the dissension and often vicious conflicts between factions in the profession.

Histories of conventional medicine, on the other hand, have been written without reference to some of its more shameful and embarrassing facets. One can celebrate orthodox medicine without pointing out that Harvey was ridiculed for saying that the blood circulates, or that Semmelweis was committed to an asylum for trying to prevent infection during surgery, or the politics involving the two competing polio vaccines, etc. But one cannot really ignore the contentious aspects of naturopathic medicine because it is populated by contentious people.

The profession is now at a point in its history that echoes that of the osteopaths a century ago. The progressives in that field wanted a different curriculum in their schools, higher academic standards, and a scope of practice that incorporated the drugs and surgery of regular medicine. Traditionalists wanted to remain a joint-manipulating, drugless profession. Their civil war did not last long. Osteopathy gave way to osteopathic medicine. Today, DOs are nearly indistinguishable from MDs and the majority of osteopathic doctors do not use any manual treatment at all. The chiropractor has taken the place of the traditional osteopath in American culture.

As naturopathic medicine replaces traditional Naturopathy, and the new breed increasingly uses mainstream medical techniques, some exclusionary tactics have been used to eliminate more traditional practitioners from the marketplace. The battle is *said to be* about academic standards and consumer protection but from an insider's point of view, these are not the true issues. It is simply the differing vision of a group that has grown to size and power and can insist that its image of the profession is the "correct" one. By becoming more compatible with (and more similar to) conventional physicians, this group is asserting its place in the health care system and is increasingly the "face" of the naturopathic doctor in the United States.

Things are different elsewhere in the world, however. I regret that with few exceptions, I was not able to write extensively about naturopathic history in other countries, except where a particular event was pertinent for that year or period. The book should probably be called *A Century of Naturopathy in America*. It is my hope that someone will pick up the spear and that I can look forward to reading in the future *A Century of Naturopathy in England* and *A Century of Naturopathy in Germany*, etc.

In the meantime, I hope my colleagues enjoy seeing their predecessors in this book and possibly pick up a new fact or two.

I end with the typical closing used by that giant of Naturopathy, Dr. Frederick Collins:

Vigorously yours,

C.P. Negri, OMD, NMD
2010

DEDICATION

To the memory of

DR. NORMAN M. ABBE

My mentor

1

ORIGINS

Hippocrates wrote extensively of the baths and moist packs that were applied to treat wounds and fevers around 450 BCE. His followers were required to learn massage as well, creating what is likely the very foundation for future development of natural medicine. Hippocrates was the first to create a *system* of medicine, and the methods he used were to be practiced from then on.

Ancient Rome also had its healing uses of water. The slave Antonius Musa cured the emperor Augustus using water applications, and also the emperor's much loved Horatio, who suffered what would later be called a nervous breakdown.

Hippocrates' reliance on water was taken up later by Aelius Galenus, better known as Galen. In 145 CE, he began the study of the healing art, and later introduced the use of oral medicines, as well as the concepts of diagnosis and prognosis, which made him effectively the seed-planter of what would become conventional medicine. Later, however, the great Swiss physician Paracelsus would restore the water treatments of Hippocrates, and the use of non-drug agents again came to prominence.

In the 18th Century, those following the Galenic form of medicine found themselves directly opposed by a new system: *Homeopathy*. Dr. Samuel Hahnemann in Germany proposed a new way of using oral medicines, and emphasized that hygiene, dietary regulation--and even applications of water--were important.

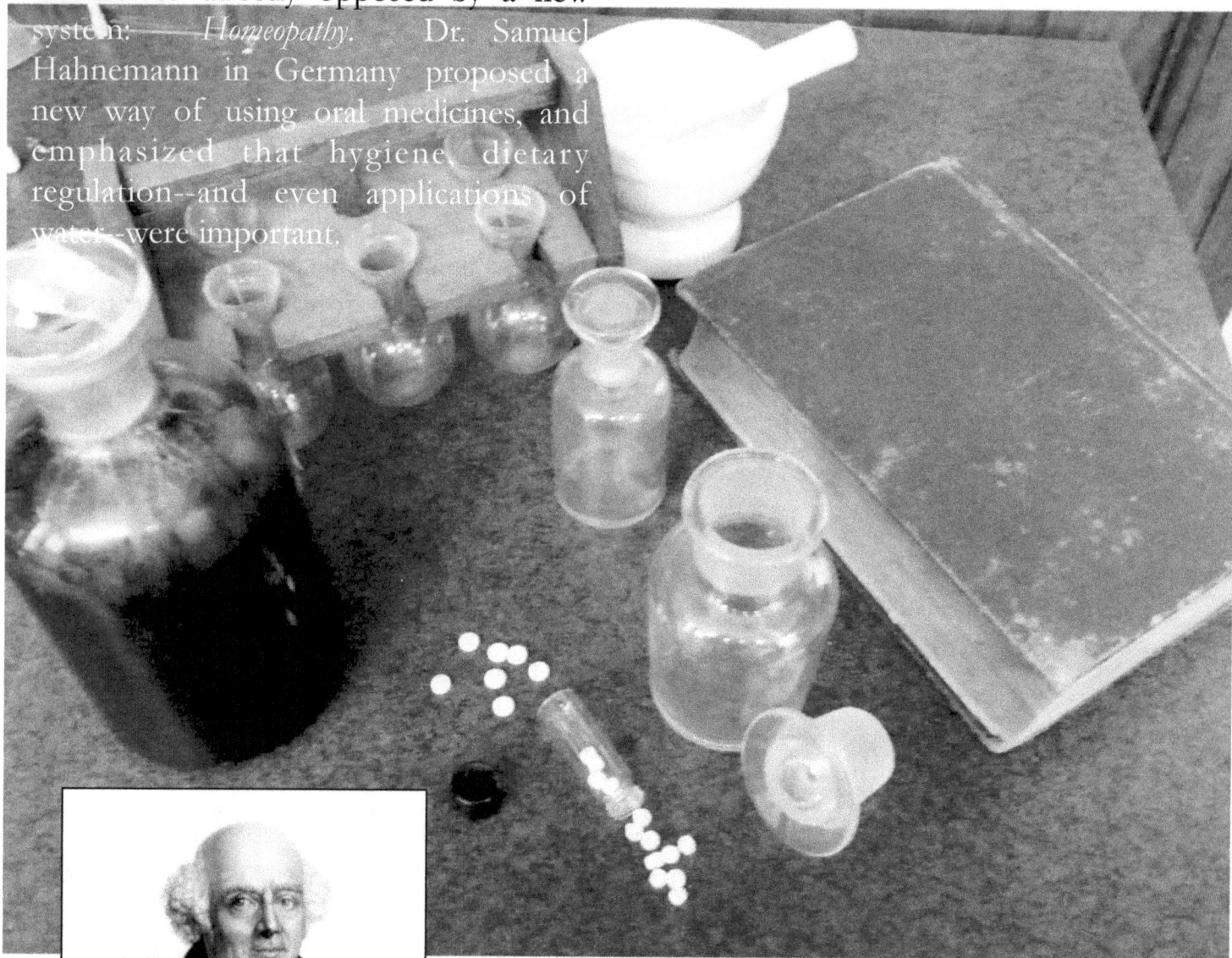

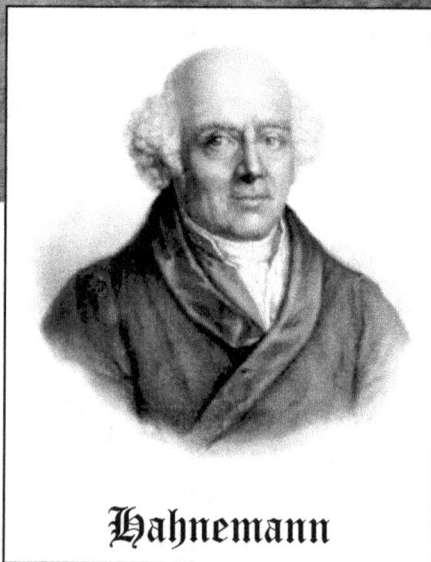

Hahnemann

Throughout the next century, war would be waged between the regular school of medicine and homeopathic medicine over what constituted effective oral agents.

While the two camps argued over pills, another type of doctor was emerging; a throwback to earlier times.

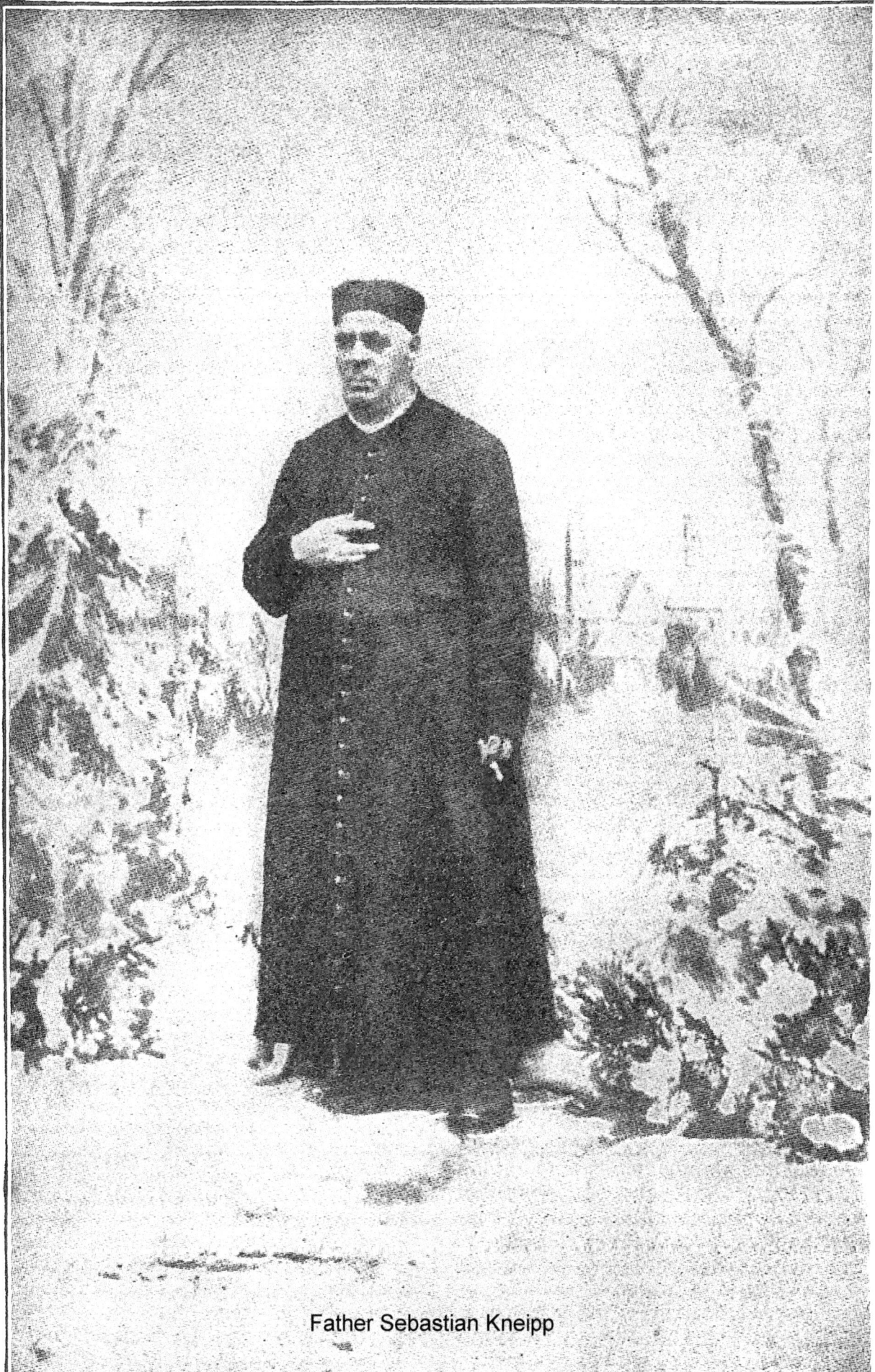

Father Sebastian Kneipp

Germany

- **Johann Sigismund Hahn** (1696-1773) of Silesia, Austria, follows in his father Sigmund's footsteps in treating disease with hydrotherapy. The elder Hahn sought to restore water cure methods from Hippocrates' time, having demonstrated the efficacy of hydrotherapy during an epidemic of petechial fever in 1737. But the son became more prominent and associated with the practice. He probably influenced, directly or indirectly, all the nature cure practitioners to follow.

1818—

- **Vincent Preissnitz** of Graefenburg in the Austrian Tyrol establishes a healing practice using hydrotherapy and diet.

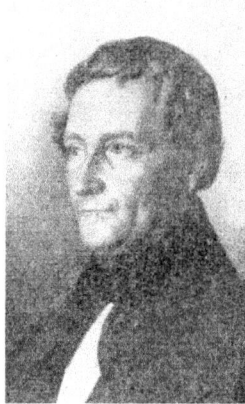

1838—

- **J.H. Rausse**, disciple of Preissnitz, refines those methods and writes the first book on the subject*.

- **Johann Schroth** of Prague, a contemporary of Preissnitz, originates the practice of the layered healing pack. To avoid the frequent changing of cold water packs as typically used, he placed several on top of the other and covered with a bandage, allowing a prolonged moist heat to be created, which had a more powerful effect in dissolving poisons in the tissues and carrying them away. He also used diet, fasting, and thirsting (alternating days of no liquids) to great effect.

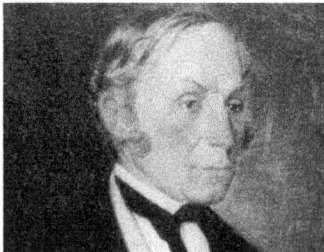

- **Lorenz Gleich** of Bavaria is the first to promote use of the term *naturarzt*, or nature doctor♦.

1854—

- **Fr. Sebastian Kneipp** of Bavaria simplifies hydrotherapy and uses it along with herbal medicines and diet to cure thousands over the next forty years. If Johann Hahn laid the foundation for modern hydrotherapeutics and Preissnitz developed it, Kneipp refined it and systematized it. His name would still be famous in Europe a hundred years after his death. †

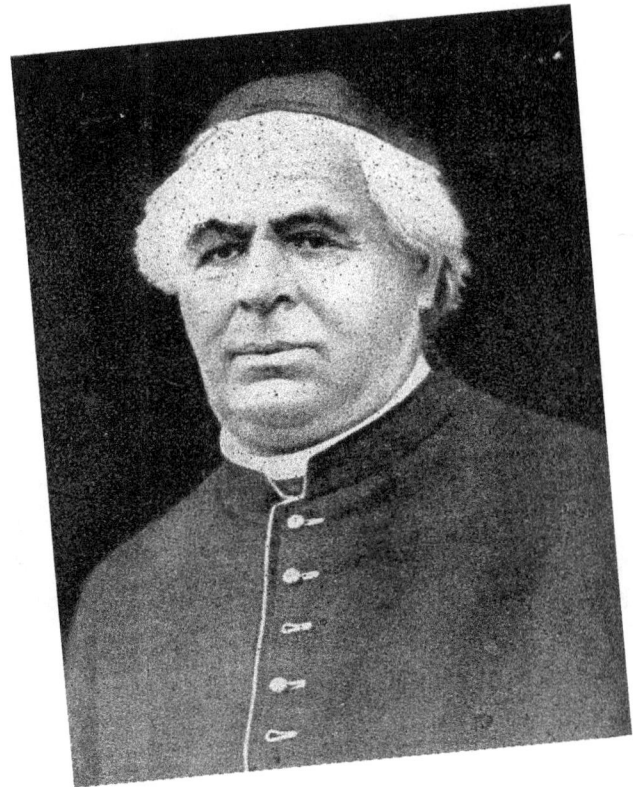

* *Naturopath and Herald of Health*, Mar. 1937, p. 90

♦ Rothschuh KE, The conceptualization of hydrotherapy in the 19th century. J. H. Rausse, Theodor Hahn, Lorenz Gleich, Gesnerus. 1981;38(1-2):175-90. PMID: 7014376 [PubMed - indexed for MEDLINE]

† Kirchfeld, Friedhelm, and Wade Boyle. "Nature Doctors: Pioneers in Naturopathic Medicine". Medicina Biologica, 1994

1861—

Wilhelm Winternitz resigns his position as surgeon and establishes a practice in Vienna centered on hydrotherapy. He will be admitted to the faculty of the University of Vienna as *privat-docent* in hydrotherapy in 1865. He will open a private hospital the same year. His work will go on to inspire and influence John Harvey Kellogg in America.

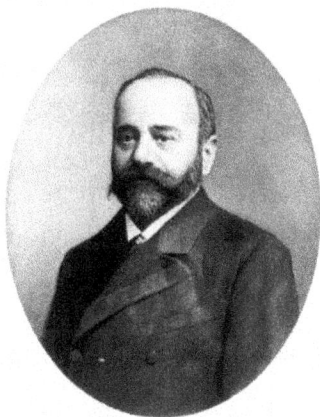

1864—

Theodor Hahn develops his own style of hydrotherapy combined with vegetarianism, and originates the term *naturheilkundt* (nature cure).

1865—

Arnold Rikli adds steam baths, air baths, and sun baths to hydrotherapy and nature cure practice. He invented new combinations of Preissnitz's water treatments and was especially influential in the concept of contrast (alternating hot and cold) treatments.

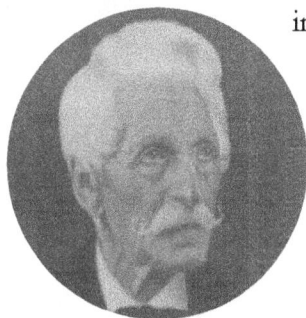

1882—

Fr. Sebastian Kneipp writes *My Water Cure*, a hydrotherapy guidebook. It will become a guide for the coming hydrotherapy movement in America, extending its influence for decades.

1883—

Louis Kuhne of Leipzig establishes the "New Science of Healing Without Drugs or Operations"; it would inspire Mahatma Gandhi to establish nature cure institutions in India.

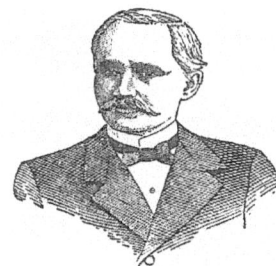

Kuhne

1888—

Heinrich Lahmann establishes an advanced nature cure sanatorium near Dresden, eventually containing 30 buildings and 350 employees. Lahmann adds constitutional typing, physical diagnosis, urinalysis, and pH balancing to nature cure methodology.

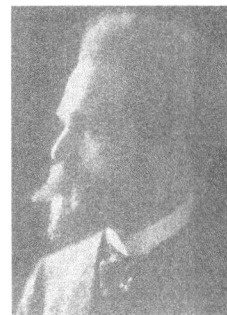

1891—

Louis Kuhne writes *The New Science of Healing*, a treatise on the basic principles of natural healing.

1892—

Freidrich E. Bilz establishes his nature cure facility, "Bilz' Natur-Heilanstalt". Located at Radebuel, Dresden; it is believed to be the largest nature cure sanatorium in the world and will be the center of the nature cure movement in Europe for years. Using virtually every type of therapy so far discovered, from diet and exercise to hydrotherapy, massage, and herbal medicines, the Natur-Heilanstalt was a magnificent complex, and some of the buildings are still in existence today.

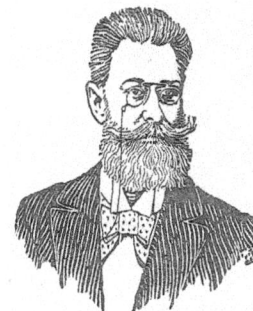

Bilz is an often neglected name in the history of natural medicine. He probably contributed more than many others to the development of what would later come to be called **Naturopathy**. Bilz wrote a masterwork of 2,000 pages, *The Natural Method of Healing*. Translated into many languages, it would be used as a major textbook in naturopathic colleges all over the world for years.

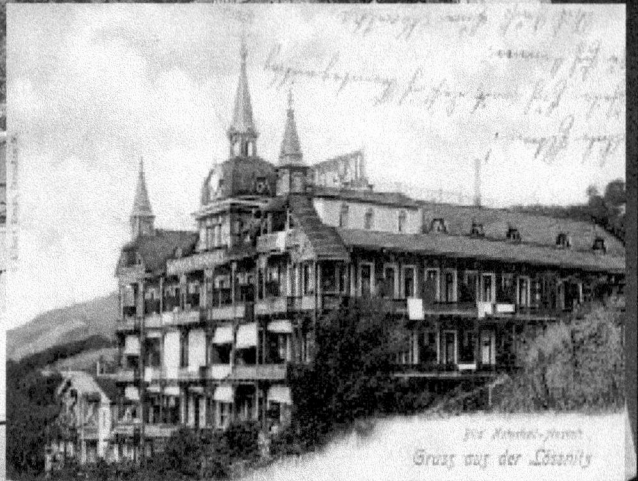

Bilz' Natur-Heilanstalt Dresden-Radebeul.

Sanatorium I. Ranges.

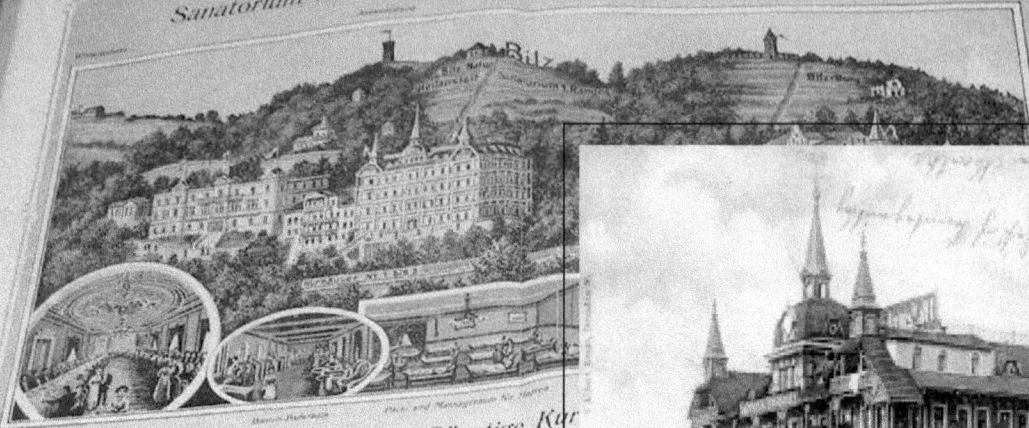

3 Anstalts-Aerzte. Günstige Kur

Bilz Natur-heilanstalt

ATLAS
äußerer und innerer
Krankheiten
des
menschlichen Körpers
zu
Bilz.Naturheilverfahren.

In 146 Einzeldarstellungen
auf 18 Tafeln abgebildet

LEIPZIG
F. E. Bilz.

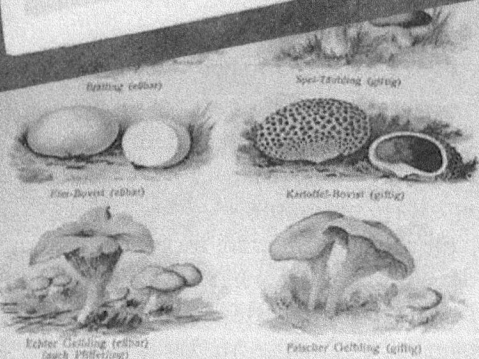

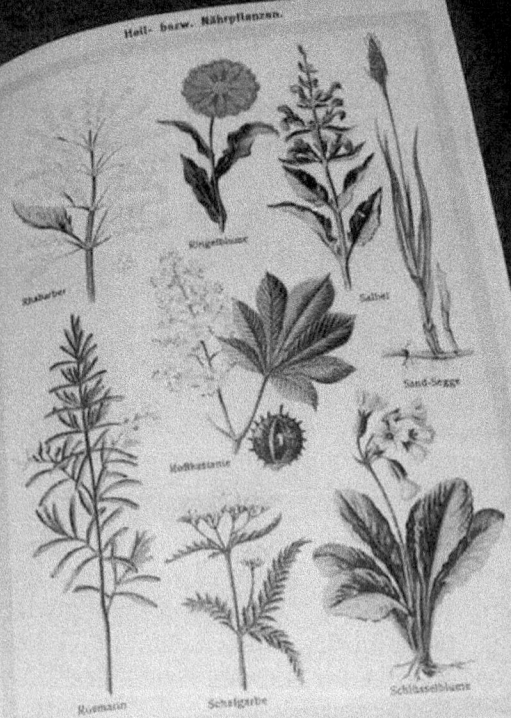

1894—

- **Emanuel Felke** adds homeopathic remedies, clay baths, and iris diagnosis to nature cure methodology. He establishes two nature cure sanatoriums, at Repellen and Sobernheim.

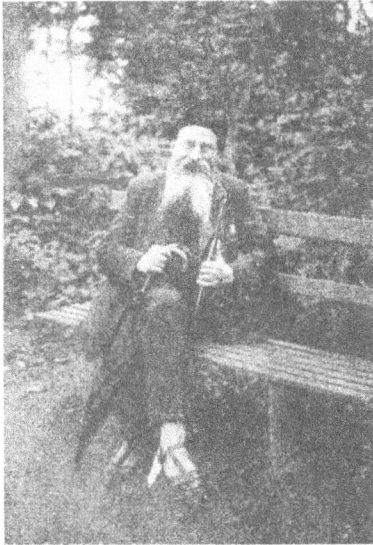

The use of clay and mineral-rich sand immersion became a popular therapy not only in Germany but on the other side of the world, in Japan.

1896—

- **Adolph Just** of the Hartz Mountains establishes a nature cure sanatorium in North Germany; and writes *Return to Nature*.

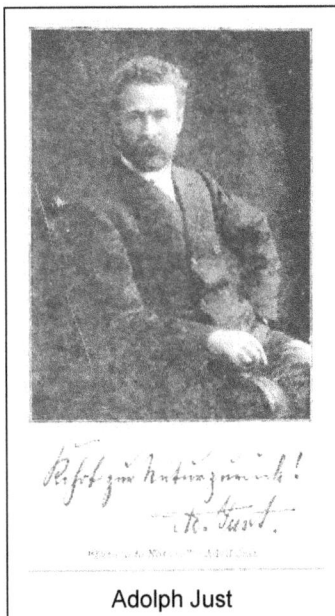

Adolph Just

1896—

- **Benedict Lust** is sanctioned by Fr. Kneipp to bring nature cure to America. He settles in New York City and establishes the Lust-Regeniter College, a Kneipp method water cure establishment.

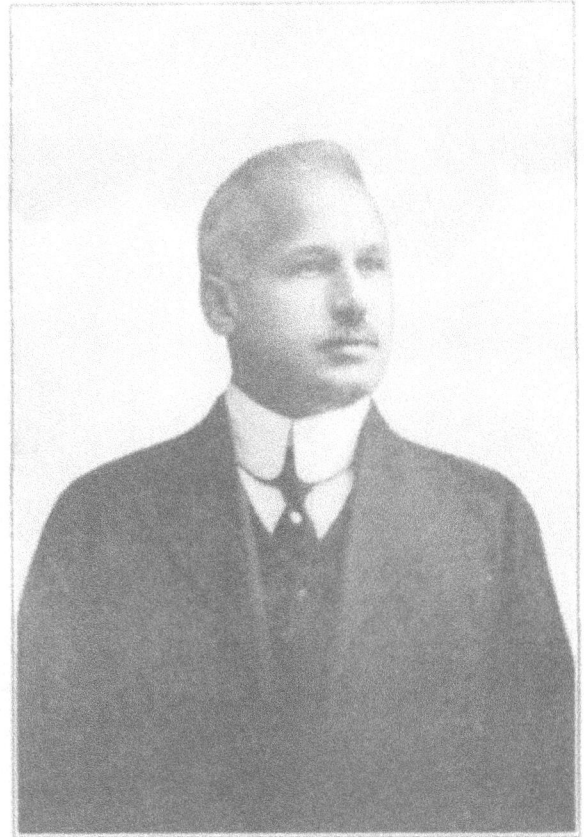

1897—

Father Kneipp dies. His name will be just as well known in Germany, and as synonymous with healing, a hundred years in the future.

1900—

Ernst Schweininger establishes the first nature cure inpatient hospital in the world, at Gross-Lichterfelde (near Berlin).

2

NEW CENTURY,
NEW MEDICINE

THE TREE OF TOXEMIA
IN THE SOIL OF
HUMAN HABITS AND BEHAVIOR

Dr. Lindlahr's Sanitarium for Nature Cure
Our Beautiful Home of Nature Cure

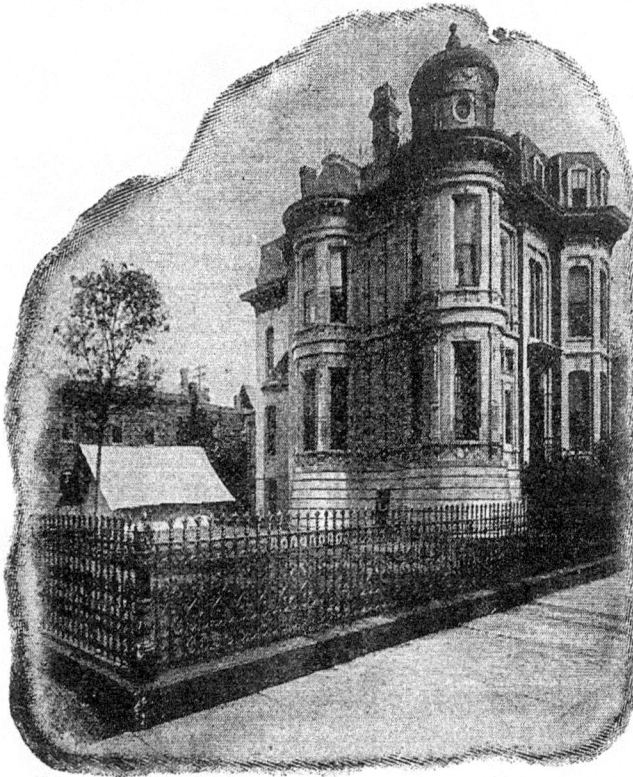

offers complete sanitarium facilities to patients from a distance and to those who wish to live the natural life in natural surroundings. We successfully treat all forms of so-called incurable diseases without the use of poisonous drugs or surgery.

NATURE CURE BY MAIL. In this department we are prepared to take care of patients at a distance who cannot have the benefit of instruction and treatment in our sanitarium. Free literature and diagnosis blank furnished on application.

Courteous attention given to all correspondence.

Send for Valuable Free Health-Culture Literature.

A LIMITED NUMBER OF VOLS. I. and II. of the NATURE CURE MAGAZINE, cloth bound, are now for sale. Price $1.50 per volume, postpaid.

Dr. Lindlahr's Sanitarium

525 Ashland Boulevard, Chicago,   Telephone, Monroe 2246

Down town offices and Treatment rooms: 84 Adams St., Rooms 404-406, Telephone Harrison 6130

AMERICA

1901—

Benedict Lust, armed with his training under Father Kneipp, attends the New York Homeopathic Medical College and graduates in 1901. He is ridiculed for his preoccupation with hydrotherapy and diet. He obtains a second degree in 1902 from the Universal College of Osteopathy in New York.

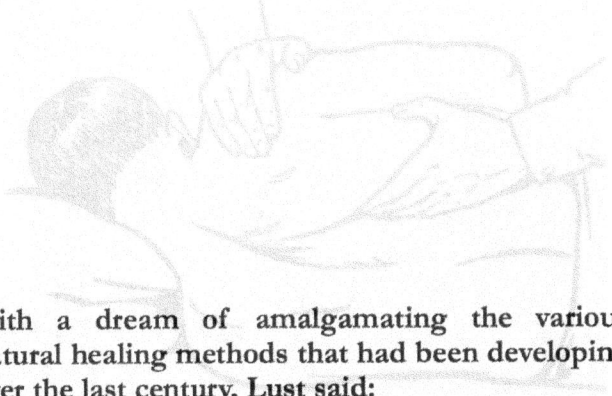

With a dream of amalgamating the various natural healing methods that had been developing over the last century, Lust said:

"The natural system for curing disease is based on a return to Nature in regulating the diet, breathing, exercising, bathing, and the employment of various forces to eliminate the poisonous products in the system, and so raise the vitality of the patient to a proper standard of health."

1902—

• **Dr. John Scheel and Dr. Sophie Scheel (a homeopathic physician) coin the term** *Naturopathy* to describe the amalgamation of natural therapies as proposed by their friend Dr. Benedict Lust, and sell the rights to the name to him. Lust announces to his circle of colleagues, "Now we have a name for our work!"

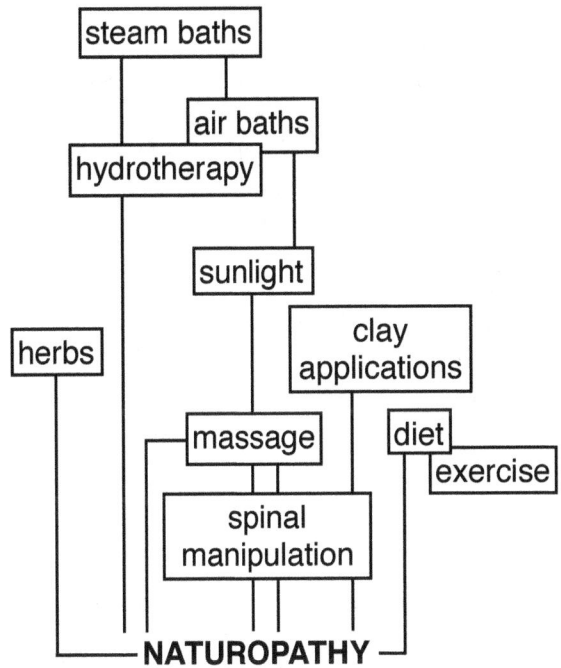

steam baths — air baths — hydrotherapy — sunlight — clay applications — herbs — massage — diet — exercise — spinal manipulation — **NATUROPATHY**

"Pathological monism and therapeutic universalism"

--Naturopathy as defined by Benedict Lust

The role of natural medicine as envisioned by Lust was "assisting Nature to remove an accumulation of morbid material in the body". Any method or device that accomplished this was acceptable; in fact, it was considered to be within the realm of Naturopathy.

1902—

- No sooner does the field have a name than it spans the continent. **Dr. Carl Schultz, "Father of Naturopathy on the West Coast", organizes the Association of Naturopathic Physicians of California.** Like Lust, Schultz trained in Germany.

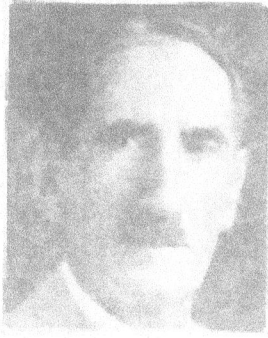

- **Benedict Lust establishes the American School of Naturopathy in New York City,** the first naturopathic school in the U.S. Originally located at 135 E. 58th St., it periodically outgrows its facilities and moves several times throughout its histor⁓

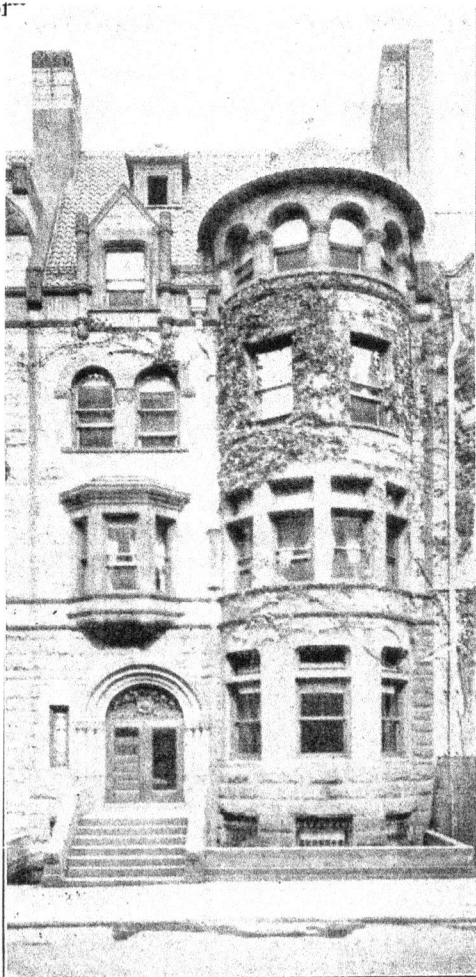

American School of Naturopathy

- **Bernarr MacFadden's** *Physical Culture* Magazine has been spreading the philosophy of "physcultopathy" to the masses. Benedict Lust declares MacFadden's methods to be part of Naturopathy, and welcomes him into the fold. MacFadden would become a member and supporter of many naturopathic organizations.

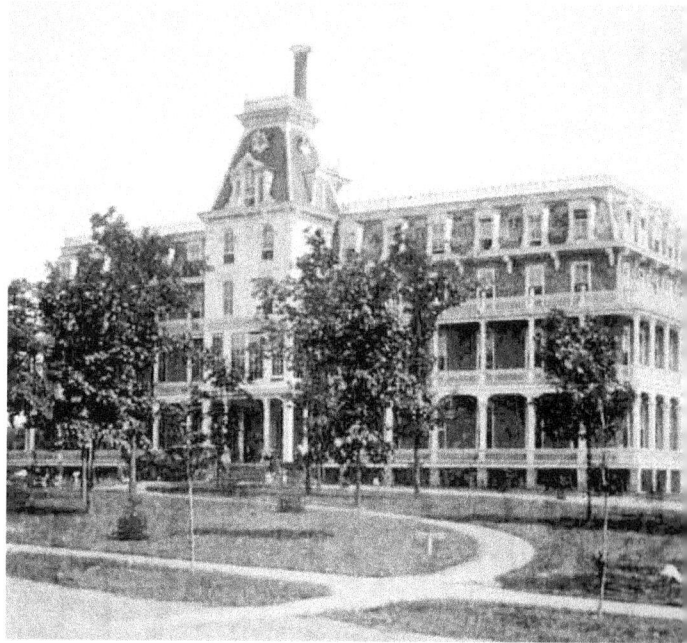

- **The Western Health Reform Institute** (above) in Michigan burns down in 1902. It will be rebuilt as the **Battle Creek Sanitarium,** and under the direction of Dr. John Harvey Kellogg, will offer inpatient treatment utilizing nearly every known modality of natural medicine. Kellogg would particularly use and refine methods of hydrotherapy that had passed down from Preissnitz and Kneipp. Two entire buildings of the new complex would be devoted to water treatments.

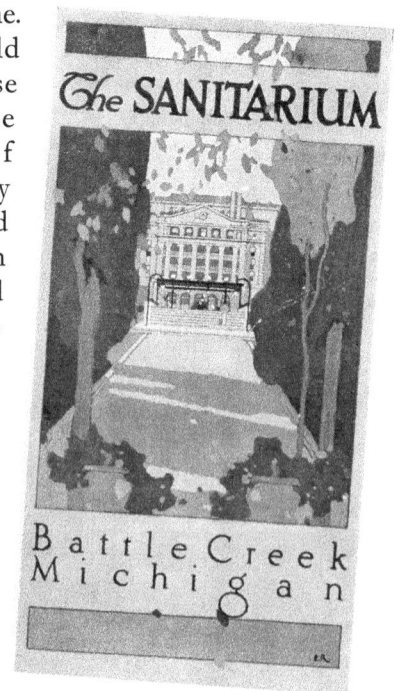

The SANITARIUM

Battle Creek Michigan

1903 —

- **Dr. F.E. Bilz dies.** Bilz, who ran a sanatorium in Dresden-Radebuel, Germany, authored the first Nature Cure encyclopedia, *Bilz, das Neue Naturheilverfahren* (The Natural Method of Healing). The two-volume, 2,000-page textbook was a comprehensive guide to natural medicine and contained much anatomical and physiological information at a time when medical textbooks were restricted. Many color guides to different pathologies and healing plants, etc., were included.

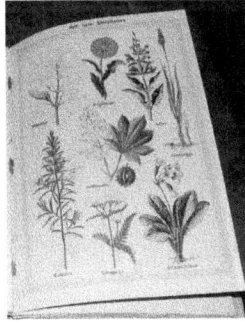

1904 —

- **Naturopathic Institute, Sanatorium, and College established** in Los Angeles by Dr. Carl Schultz. It is the second institution to use the term "naturopathic". Schultz's Naturopathic Institute would be the wellspring for naturopathic education on the west coast.

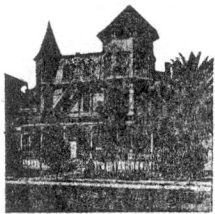

THE
20th Century
Method of Regaining
LOST HEALTH

NATUROPATHY

Naturopathy is to-day restoring vigor and vim to those suffering from run-down, debilitated conditions of the system when drugs fail to have any effect. Our fees are exceedingly reasonable and outside patients may come and take treatment between the hours of 8 to 12 a.m. and 2 to 8 p.m. Treatment consists of

Naturopathy is the Natural Way of Treating Disease

MASSAGE, OSTEOPATHY, CHIROPRACTIC, SPONDYLOTHERAPY, ORTHOPEDIC SURGERY, SUGGESTION, HYDROTHERAPY in all branches, ELECTRIC LIGHT, HOT AIR, VAPOR, SUN, HERBAL, PINE NEEDLE, NAUHEIM and all other MEDICATED BATHS, OUR TREATMENT ROOMS AND ROOMS FOR RESIDENT PATIENTS ARE SUNNY AND STEAM HEATED.

Naturopathic Institute and Sanitorium
OF CALIFORNIA (Incorporated)
DR. CARL SCHULTZ, President
1319 S. GRAND AVENUE   LOS ANGELES, CAL.
Phones: Home 20903; Broadway 2707

- **Dr. Benedict Lust translates** and publishes the first English edition of Adolph Just's book, *Return To Nature*.

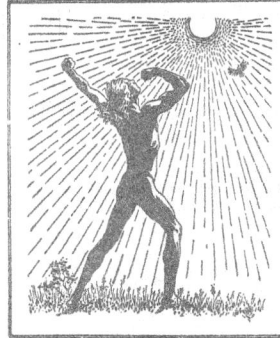

RETURN
TO
NATURE

By

ADOLF JUST

Considered by many authorities the pre-eminent book (for the layman) on Nature Cure, we unhesitatingly state that we believe more people have been converted to natural living by this work than any similar book. Simplicity itself, it deals with Nature from the spiritual, mental and physical points of view in the most convincing manner. Sun, air, water, earth, food, all the forces of nature are made so clear and alive that skeptics are easily converted. This book is a vital part of every Nature Cure library. It is known as the "Bible of the Body."

- **Dr. Otto Carque begins teaching iris diagnosis,** which would become a naturopathic tool.

Still, no naturopathic institution--at least one using the word "naturopathic"--matched the fame or grandeur of the massive Battle Creek Sanitarium. Within its four main buildings, treatments could be administered to up to a thousand patients, four hundred of whom could be lodged there. Kellogg described the system there as "a complete physiologic method comprising hydrotherapy, phototherapy, thermotherapy, electrotherapy, mechanotherapy, dietetics, physical culture, cold air cure, and health training." With over 30 doctors in attendance, the most up-to-date medical diagnostic methods were used, but the treatments were drawn from Naturopathy. Kellogg was one of a number of conventionally-trained medical doctors who used natural therapeutics but did not call themselves naturopaths.

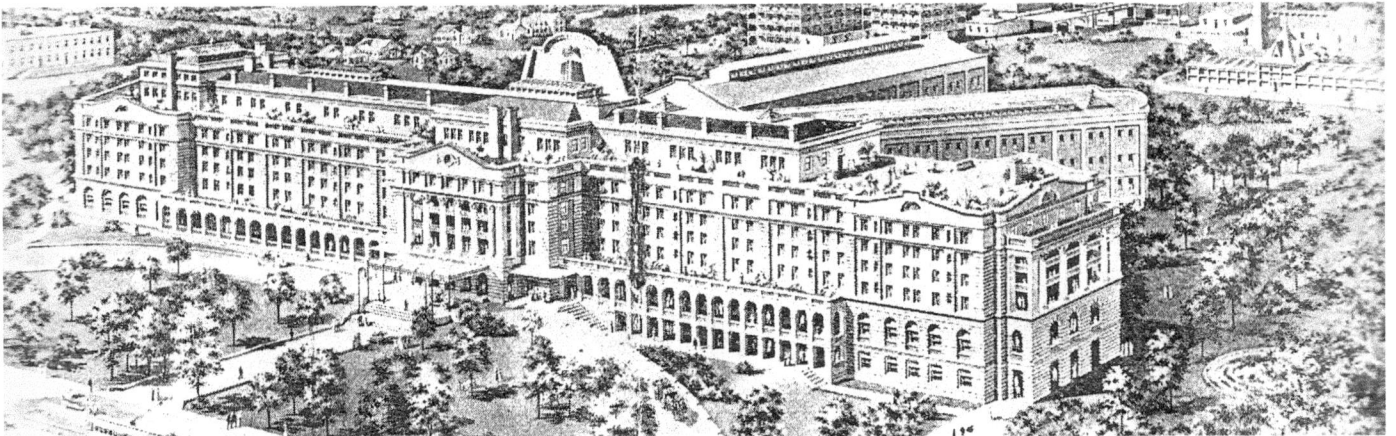

Battle Creek Sanitarium

1906—

- **Dr. Henry Lindlahr establishes the Sanitarium of Nature Cure** in Chicago. A second facility will be located in rural Elmhurst, Illinois. Lindlahr will refer to his method as "natural therapeutics", rather than the more sectarian-sounding "Naturopathy".

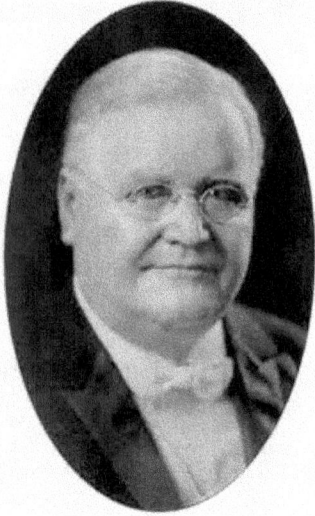

Henry Lindlahr, M.D.

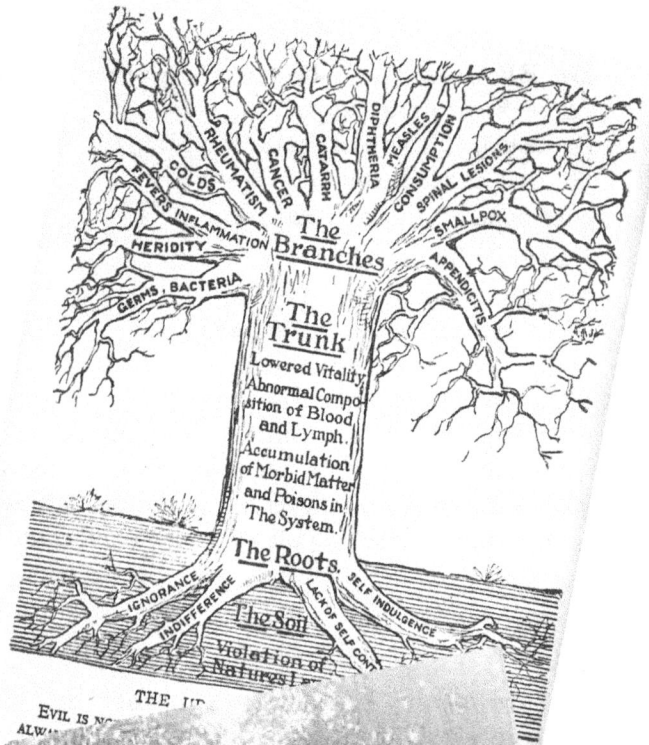

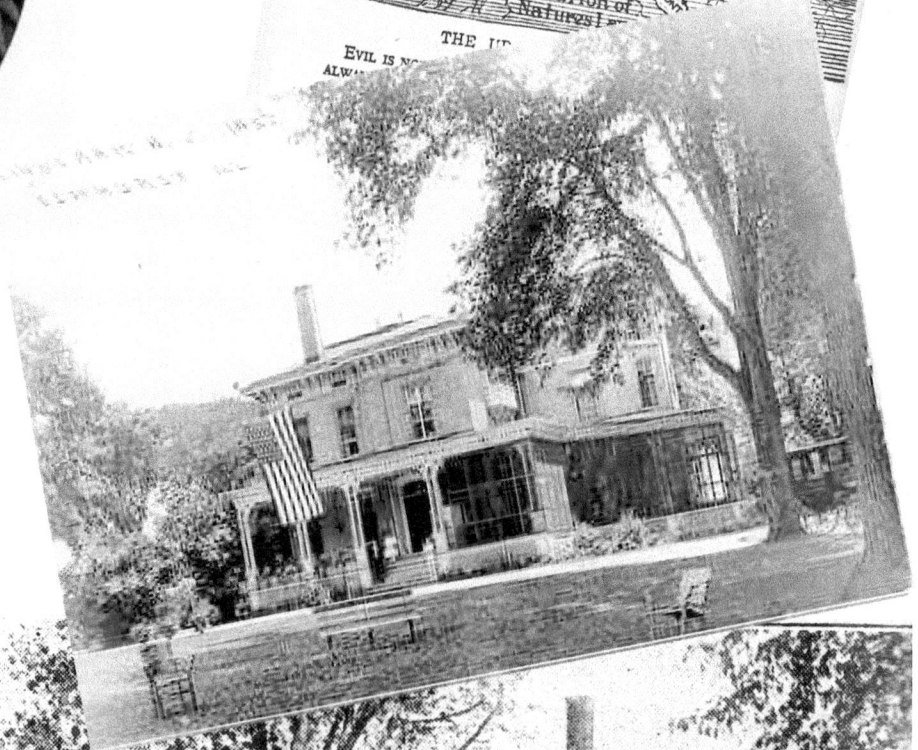

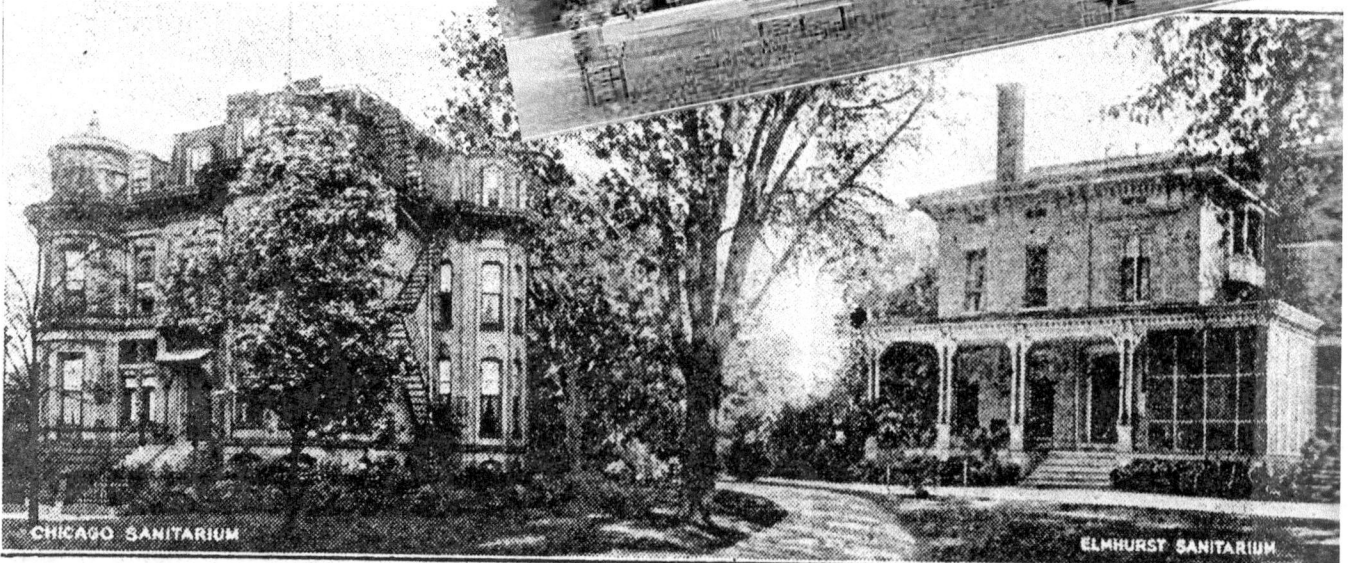

CHICAGO SANITARIUM

ELMHURST SANITARIUM

A success from its inception, Lindlahr's sanitarium would grow to two locations, then expanding to serve the growing number of patients conventional medicine failed. Note the various therapies used: Homeopathy, Hydrotherapy, Osteopathy, Physiotherapy, etc. Lindlahr's son Victor would succeed him in running the facilities.

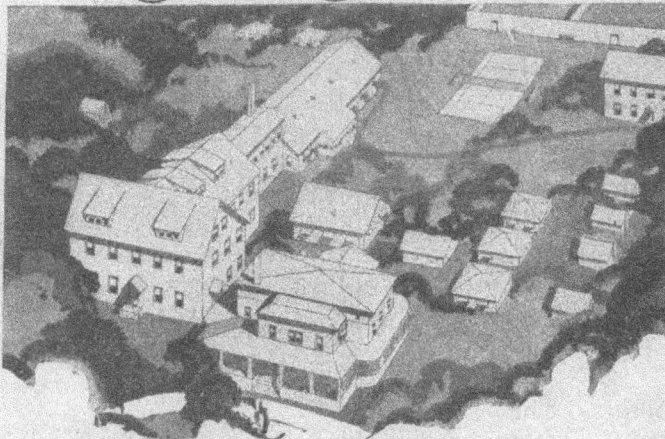

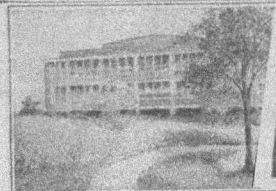

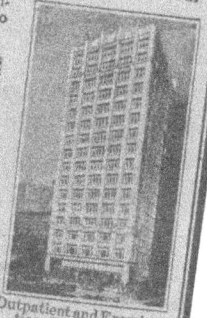

1907—

- **The Governor of California** was granted the authority to appoint eleven members to a board to regulate the practice of medicine. The board was to be composed of five allopaths, two homeopaths, two eclectics and two osteopaths. No naturopaths or chiropractors were admitted to the board. (Compare with the national panel established in 1995, Chapter 7)

- Lust's **American School of Naturopathy** acquires a building at 465 Lexington Ave., formerly a homeopathic hospital and surgical clinic. The operating rooms were converted to gymnasiums and lecture halls.

1909—

- **California licenses naturopathic doctors.** The Association of Naturopathic Physicians of California succeeds in getting a licensing bill passed.

- **Bernarr MacFadden** establishes the first naturopathic sanatorium in England, at Brighton.

- **Andrew P. Davis, MD, ND, DO, DC** creates his own system, "Neuropathy"—an integrated method like Naturopathy, containing techniques of such varied treatments as hydrotherapy, diet, magnetic healing, suggestive therapeutics, and even ophthalmology. The dominant techniques used, however, are drawn from Osteopathy and Chiropractic. In this year he publishes his major work, *Neuropathy: The New Science of Drugless Healing Amply Illustrated and Explained.* He established the Davis College of Neuropathy in Los Angeles. Some prominent naturopaths of later years, such as Thomas T. Lake, ND, would have instruction there.

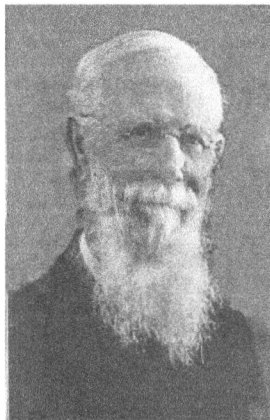

1910—

- **Elmer Lee, MD**, converts to naturopathic practice and establishes a movement called "The Hygienic System". He publishes a periodical called *Health Culture* for many years.

- **Dr. Frederick W. Collins** establishes the **United States School of Naturopathy** in New Jersey. It will go on to become one of the colleges in the expanded First National University of Therapeutics, along with an osteopathic college, a chiropractic college, and a school of physical therapy.

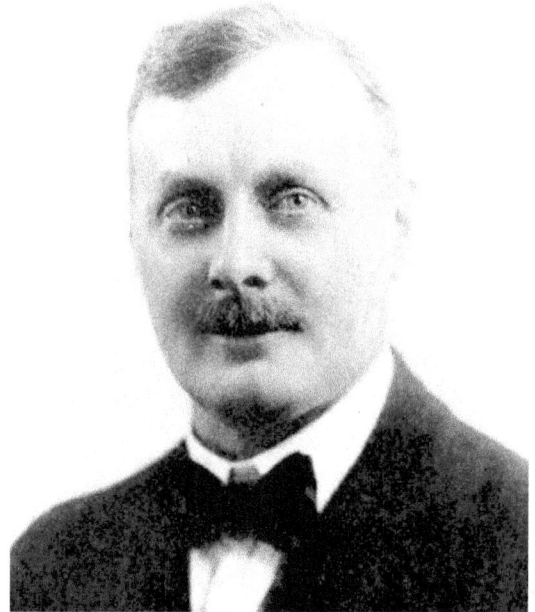

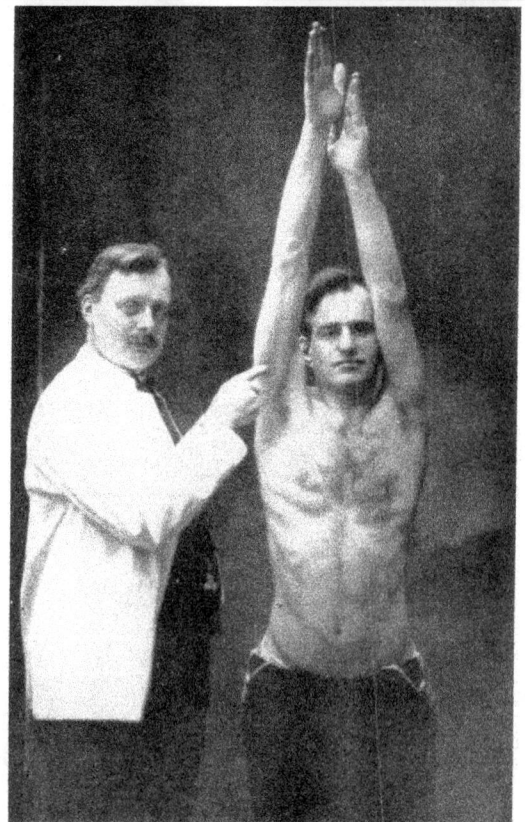

16

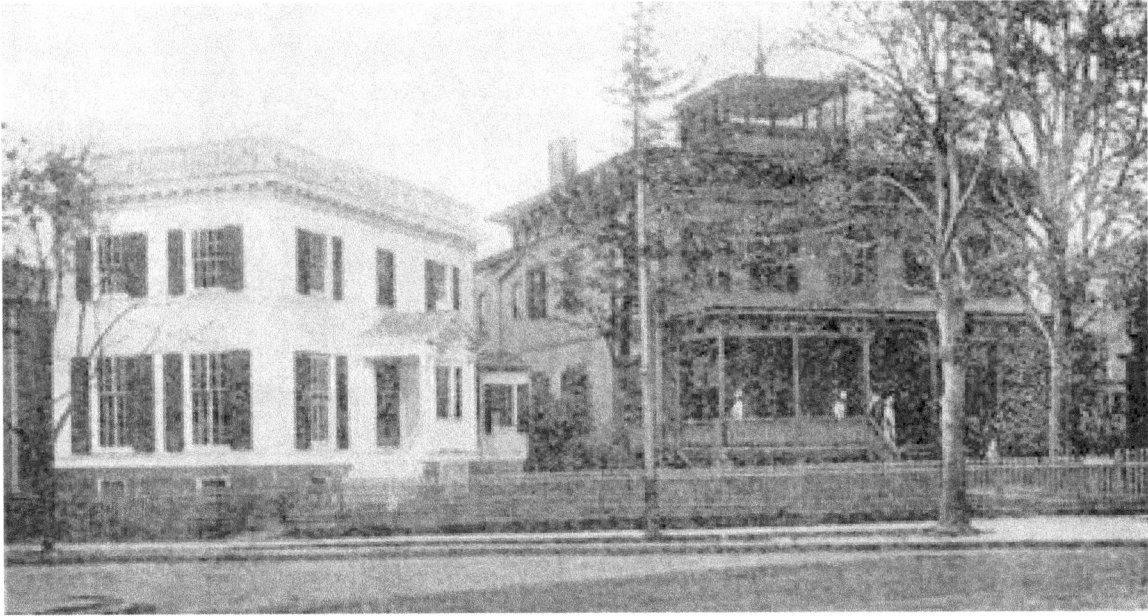

Campus, First National University
United States School of Naturopathy

- *Brain And Brawn,* a new naturopathic journal out of Los Angeles, joins Benedict Lust's *The Naturopath and Herald of Health* in disseminating information to the profession and the public alike. Harry Ellington Brook, ND, is editor. Its philosophy: "A Sound Mind in a Sound Body". "Devoted to the Nature Cure," it proclaimed, and was another sign that the west coast naturopathic movement was growing.

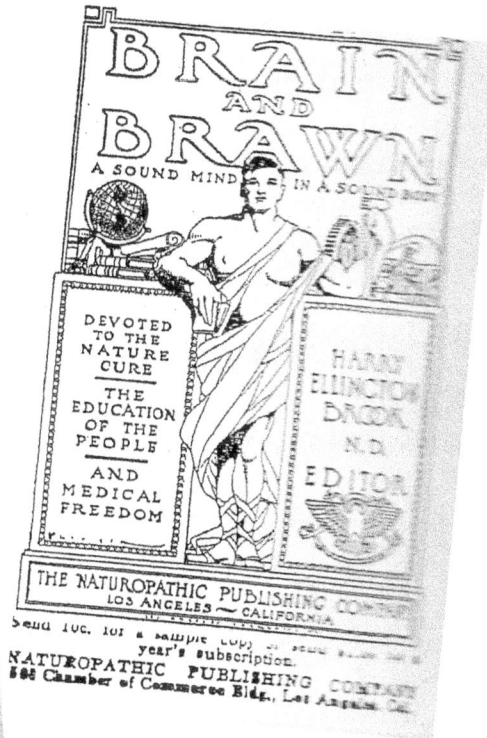

Toxemia Explained

By Dr. J. H. TILDEN

A BOOK fully explaining what Dr. Tilden means by the word "Toxemia." The meaning is not what you will find in the dictionaries, lexicons, thesauruses, encyclopedias, as up to date. Your language teachers will not know unless they are traveling faster than "standard" living "English authors," the dead ones would have lived longer if they had known the larger meaning read into it by Dr. Tilden.

"Toxemia Explained"
$2.00 Postpaid

"Toxemia Explained," with the periodical, "Tilden Health Review & Critique," for one year, $3.00.

Address

P. O. Box 1677, Denver, Colorado

17

1913—

Dr. Henry Lindlahr publishes *Nature Cure*, a textbook for naturopathic practice that will endure for decades. It will see print in several volumes and versions, such as *Philosophy of Natural Therapeutics*, *The Practice of Natural Therapeutics*, *Natural Therapeutics: Dietetics*, and *Natural Therapeutics: Iridiagnosis*.

1915—

John H. Tilden, MD, operates a natural therapeutics sanitarium in Denver, Colorado, which becomes as renowned in the Rockies as Lindlahr's Illinois institutions are. Tilden was an Eclectic physician, a graduate of Eclectic Institute of Cincinnati. He began to question the use of medicine during his early practice in Illinois and abandoned its use altogether, using detoxification, diet, and other natural therapies. He would establish an addition to his sanitarium, a school to teach natural therapeutics to other doctors. There was strong opposition from the regular medical establishment.

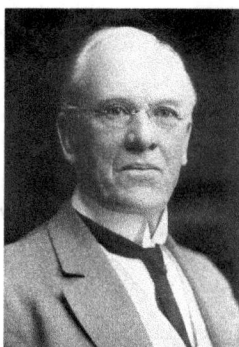

Dr. Tilden

His monthly newsletter, called *A Stuffed Club*, in print since 1900, was a forum in which Tilden espoused his philosophy of healthy living and answered questions submitted to him. In this year, 1915, its name would change to *The Philosophy of Health*. In the 1920s, he would write the book *Toxemia Explained*, which would be used for decades within the naturopathic field. He would also write *Practical Cook Book* (a food combining text); *Impaired Health, Its Cause and Cure*, Volumes I and II; *Pocket Dietician*; *Tumors—The Cause*, and others.

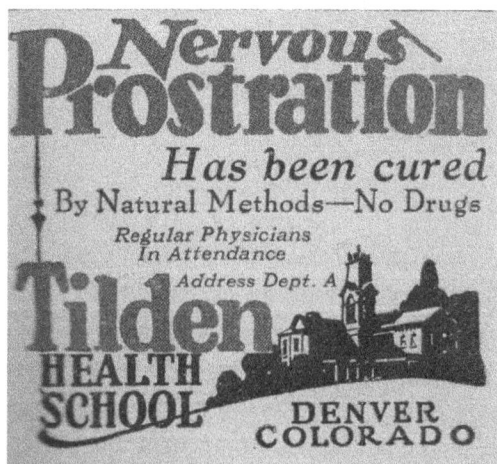

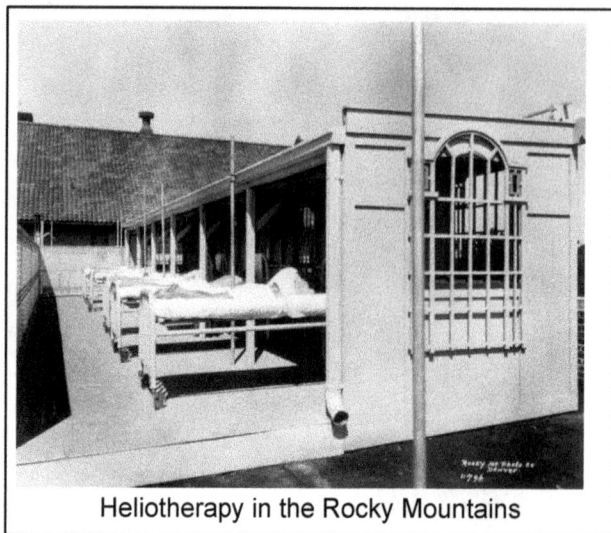

Heliotherapy in the Rocky Mountains

1917—

Benedict Lust translates and publishes Louis Kuhne's book, *Neo-Naturopathy: The New Science of Healing*.

1918—

Benedict Lust publishes the *Universal Naturopathic Encyclopedia*, a massive collection containing: a directory of drugless therapists; biographies of drugless pioneers (including Still and Palmer; founders, respectively, of Osteopathy and Chiropractic); a book and periodical guide as well as book reviews; and lists of schools and sanitariums.

It also contained articles by Lust himself, **Henry Lindlahr, MD** ("How I Became Acquainted With Nature Cure"), **Harry Ellington Brook, ND** ("Naturopathy"), **J. Allen Pattreiouex, ND** ("The Present Position Of Naturopathy And Allied Therapeutic Measures In The British Isles"), **Per Nelson, ND** (Why All Drugless Methods?"), and **Edward Earle Purinton** (Efficiency in Drugless Healing"), and **Carl Strueh, MD, ND** ("The Nature Cure"). Strueh was a comrade of Lust's during this time, and Lust referred to him as "… one of the first medical men in this country who gave up medicine and operations for natural healing."

The elaborate compilation also contained Lust's translation of **Louis Kuhne's** *Neo-Naturopathy: The New Science of Healing*, from the previous year.

"This, then, completes Volume 1 of the Naturopathic Directory, Drugless Yearbook and Buyer's Guide for the years 1918 and 1919.

"Into it, has been placed the conscientious labor of many willing hearts, hands and minds. It is their contribution to the noble cause of natural healing. It will stand as a monument to their endeavors, as well as a memorial to the great souls, the fathers of natural healing, who have passed on.

"Let this, then, herald a new era – the era wherein man shall recognize the omniscience of Nature, and shall profit through conforming to her laws."

--Conclusion to the *Universal Naturopathic Encyclopedia*

1919—

- **The American Naturopathic Association is founded by Dr. Benedict Lust,** from the original "Kneipp Society" organization, and the later "Naturopathic Society of America". The ANA will be the major unifying body for the profession for decades to come.

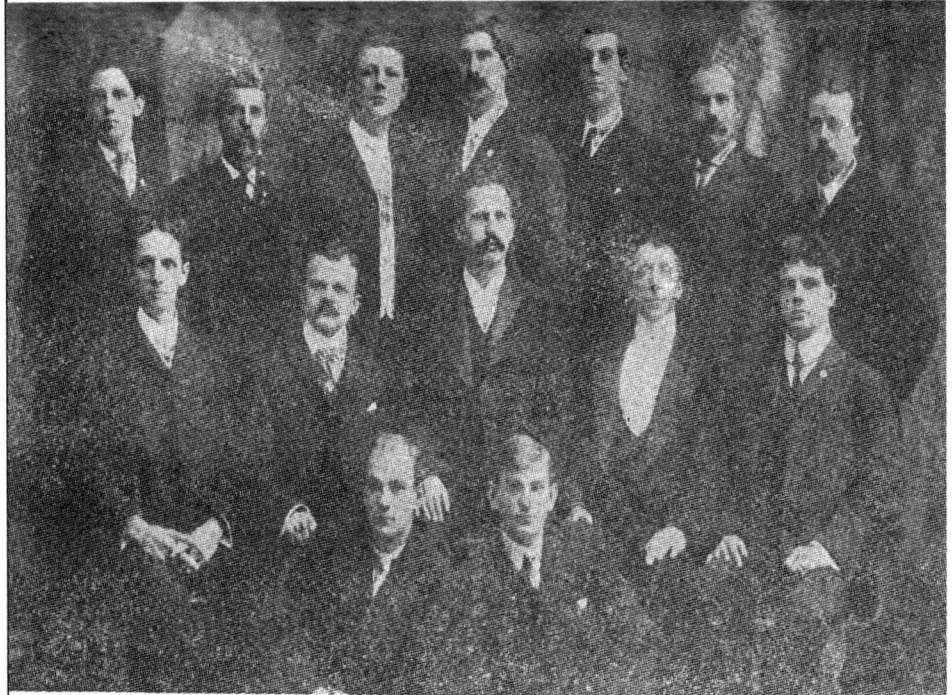

Original Members of the ANA, with Lust in the center

With Lust's motto of "therapeutic universalism", many members of the various drugless healing professions would soon come to find a home within Naturopathy. Osteopaths who loathed chiropractors, and chiropractors who disliked homeopaths, all of whom were at war with the allopaths—were welcome within the ranks of the American Naturopathic Association.

Meanwhile, elsewhere: James Thomson establishes the first four-year naturopathic college in Britain in 1919, the Edinburg School of Natural Therapeutics.

3

PROLIFERATION
AND
PROTEST

ZONE THERAPY
By Dr. BENEDICT LUST

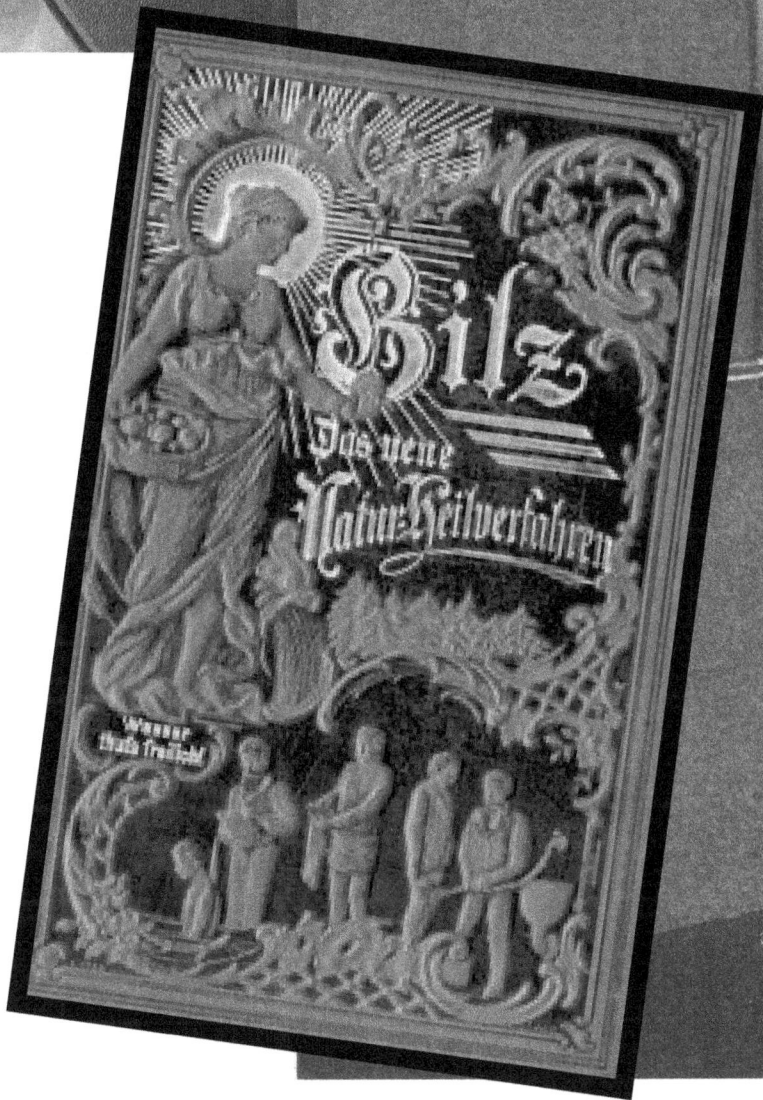

Pilz
Das neue
Natur-Heilverfahren

Naturopathy began to spread

throughout the country, as new doctors were trained on both coasts and were boldly advancing to fill the need. The public was ready.

Most Eclectic medical colleges had already closed and the homeopathic medical schools were going in the same direction. Eclectic and homeopathic medical doctors were popular with the public because their medicines were safer and they were generally more caring than the "regular" doctors, who used strong drugs, serums, and toxoids. Osteopathic doctors, once "drugless" practitioners, had turned to drugs and surgery. With Eclectic and homeopathic MDs disappearing, the only competitor to the "regular" MD was Chiropractic. While the orthodox medical community tried to portray the chiropractor as a bone-cracking quack who would never be confused with a *real* doctor, along came the naturopath.

With an armamentarium of natural methods to cover any health care need, the ND was the "regular" doctor's worst nightmare. He could adjust spines like a chiropractor *and* prescribe a special diet. He could use water to heal *and* use plant medicines as well. All the new therapy devices being manufactured were in his hands. Infra-red, ultra-violet, electrotherapy of every type, fever cabinets--everything science had to offer was being embraced.

The ND organized public educational activities where people were introduced to natural foods, exercise, and disease prevention. He campaigned for better conditions in the workplace, and against food additives. And the word was being spread through many magazines and countless lay groups. With that swelling of public support, legislators introduced bills to license the naturopathic doctors, and the battle was on.

As the NDs became more and more organized, efforts to oppose them became more and more organized as well.

1920—

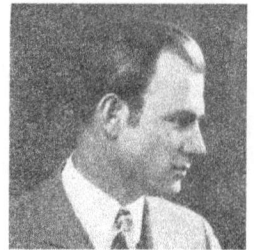

Dr. Shelton

- **Dr. Herbert Shelton** publishes his textbook, *Fundamentals of Nature Cure.*

- **An irregular group of ANA members** led by Dr. Louis Blumer establish the practice of **"Natureopathy"** in Connecticut. In order to evade Benedict Lust's trademark on the term "Naturopathy" they use a different spelling.

1921—

- **The American Naturopathic Convention** is held in Washington, DC. President Harding receives officers and delegates of the ANA. Mrs. Harding was cured by a naturopath after medical doctors had given up her case.[*]

1922—

- **The Associated Naturopathic Schools and Colleges of America** (ANSCA) agency is founded, which then standardizes curricula and accredits all U.S. naturopathic schools.

- **Benedict Lust** is given a rare honor by the President of the United States, being allowed to lay a wreath on George Washington's grave.

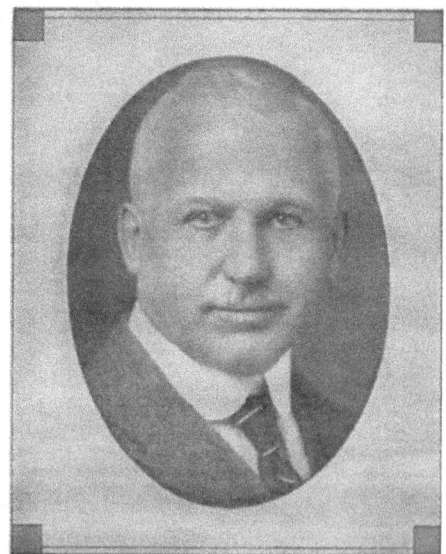

[*] *Naturopath and Herald of Health,* Jun. 1937, p. 163

Dr. Benedict Lust's reminiscences of 1922:

"At that time the medical persecution went wild that we could hold such great national conventions and had such wide recognition. The result was that the second class mail privilege was withdrawn from our publications. When I received notice I went to the head of the Second Class Mail division in New York and I asked him who was responsible for this. I was told: the medical department of the Post Office. When I asked him if these doctors who constitute the medical department in the Post office belonged to the A.M.A., he told me point blank, 'it *is* the A.M.A.' When I came to Washington and saw the authorities I was told that my magazine had been ruled out as being a danger to the public and having no educational value. Then came my hour. I told the doctor in charge that unless I got my second class mail privilege restored right then and there I would go straight to the White House and I knew a door would open for me. I told him all of our convention in the Hotel Willard. This brought the assurance that everything would be all right. When I came back to New York City the 28 bags of mail had gone out."

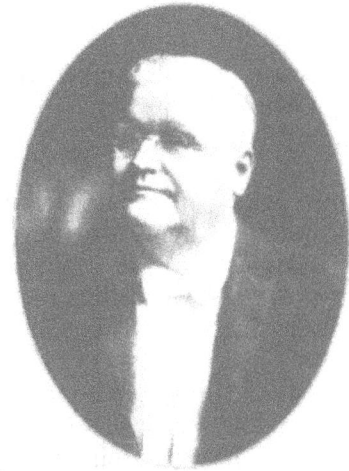

Nature's Remedies are the best.
H. Lindlahr M.D.

1923—

Connecticut licenses naturopathic doctors, using Louis Blumer's spelling, "Natureopathy".

1924—

- **Dr. Henry Lindlahr, champion of scientific natural medicine, dies.** He founded the Lindlahr College of Naturopathy in Chicago. He will always be remembered as one of the giants of natural medicine, and his most famous book, *Nature Cure, Philosophy and Practice*, still stands as the most essential text for understanding the basis of Naturopathy. As he often said, "Nature's remedies are the best." His practice and direction of his sanitariums is assumed by his son, Dr. Victor Lindlahr.

- **Herbert Shelton**, graduate of American School of Naturopathy and prolific naturopathic writer, leaves the naturopathic community to establish the more fundamentalist nature cure movement, *Natural Hygeine*. Shelton was openly critical[*] of the direction Naturopathy was going and was verbally admonished by founder Benedict Lust.

1925—

- **E.W. Cordingly, AM, ND**, writes *Principles and Practice of Naturopathy*, a textbook for the practitioner that is a "compendium of natural healing".

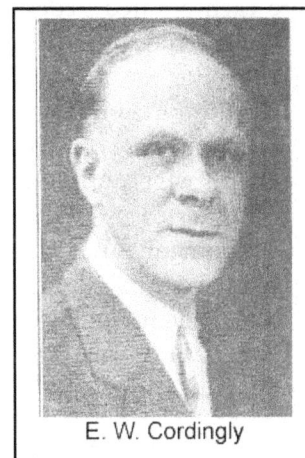

E. W. Cordingly

[*] Shelton, H., "What Have We, Nature Cure or a Bag of Tricks?" *Naturopath and Herald of Health*, (1921) 26:283-7

1925—

"Chiropractor Schools Fight Jersey Law To Ban Them" --*New York Graphic*, June 15, 1925

"The law which prevents licensing of drugless healing schools will be fought as unconstitutional to the highest court, according to Dr. F.W. Collins, dean of the United States School of Naturopathy and the Mecca School of Chiropractic, both of 143 Roseville Ave., Newark, who is free on a $200 bail pending trial June 9 on a charge of conducting a healing school without a license.

"The law which forces schools teaching healing of any kind to be licensed by the medical board is seen as a fundamental attack on drugless healing by Dr. Collins. The attitude of the medical board, he says, is that if they can stop the supply of drugless healers they can better handle the present practitioners.
"Dr. Collins declares that he will fight his case to the highest court of the country and to the last penny of his resources."

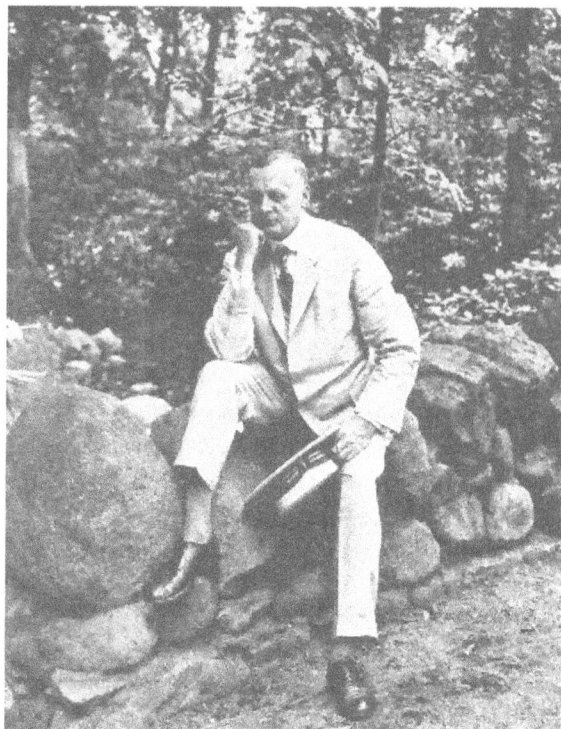

"If anybody deserves the name of 'Father of Naturopathy', it is Dr. Collins. He has done more for the cause of Naturopathy to make it known and respected than any other man living. Thanks be to him that we still have a school of Naturopathy in New Jersey. All the other schools have been closed or have been compelled to leave the state, but Dr. Collins has successfully fought every attempt made by our powerful and influential enemy the Medical Trust, the A.M.A., to close the school, and with great financial loss, kept the school open."

--Gustav G. Carlson, in a report of the School Board to the New Jersey State League of Drugless Physicians, October 1930

Although Benedict Lust was arrested many times as he fought to establish his Naturopathy as a lawful profession, no one rivaled Frederick Collins in the fight to protect natural healing. Although skirmishes in court were common during these formative days, Collins held the record for successful fights against the medical establishment. He had an extraordinary undefeated score in court cases defending Naturopathy and moreover, spent his own money to do so. Part of his success was owed to the fact that his schools were each granted Federal charters, giving them a solid validity and protection as educational institutions. Also there was a labyrinthine corporate relationship among his naturopathic school, chiropractic school, osteopathic school, and physiotherapy school, which was done deliberately to confound those seeking to use the courts to take his property in a judgment and interfere with the production of "irregular" practitioners*. Collins was a stalwart figure in the defense and development of the profession, and would be referred to in his later years as "The Dean of Naturopathy".

> There have now been up to **two dozen** schools of Naturopathy at any given time, and NDs are licensed in twenty-three states.

---

* Collins, F.W., First National University archives

24

Dr. Frederick W. Collins
The Pioneer

Respectfully dedicated by
Rev. Samuel H. Stille

Hurled from Infinite depths
By some creative power,
Robed and clothed with vigorous life
You began your so-journ here.

The quickness of lightning fills your soul,
The power of the Infinite cruises your veins,
The love of justice rules your heart,
The paths of destiny lure your feet.

In a vast un-charted jungle
It is for you to blaze a trail
To pave the way for future highways,
Replacing trails of a musty past.

You are a born fighter for the rights of men.
Keep your armor, continue the fight,
Grip the sword, enter the Courts of men,
And fight like the fighter you are.

You need not fear the hosts of wrong,
You need not fear the power of man,
For you in attune with the Infinite
Can battle a thousand men.

By and by, when it's even time,
And the stars of eternity glow,
When your spirit takes its flight
To a land beyond the hills,

You need not fear, for the race you served
Shall journey on to your high plane;
They'll pause a moment and weave a garland
And placing it whisper, "He gave his life for man."

Reprinted from *Success in the Field of Drugless Healing*, ca. 1929

1925—

- **The territory of Hawaii licenses** naturopathic doctors.

- **Louisa Lust, ND**, dies. She was the wife of the founder of Naturopathy, Benedict Lust. A nature cure practitioner even before meeting her husband, she was considered to be one of the foremost authorities on dietetics in the country.

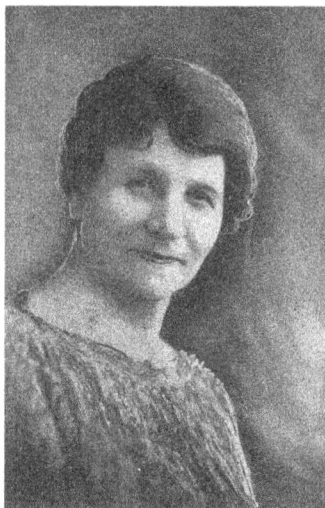

Louisa Lust, ND

Meanwhile, elsewhere...

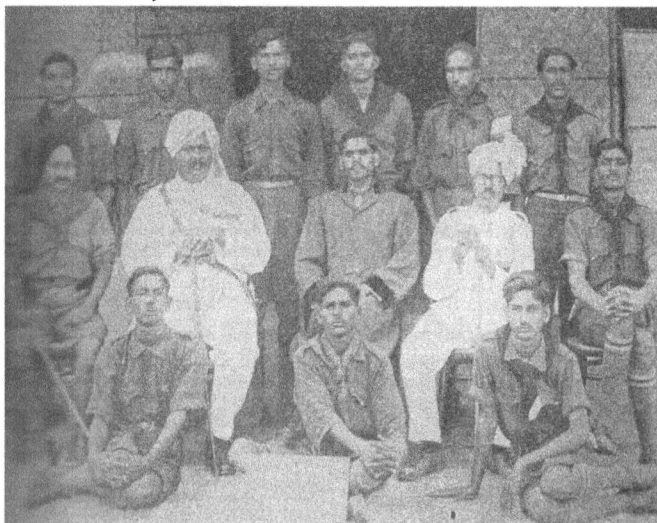

Dr. H. L. Sharma, a pioneer naturopath in India, is physician-in-charge at the Naturopathic Hospital of the Congress Volunteer Corps. He is seen in the center of the picture.

In the April 1925 issue of *The Naturopath*, G.R. Clements, ND, reports on an interesting find—C.J. Whalen, MD, writing in the *Illinois Medical Journal*, laments the growth of alternative practitioners:

"Medicine as a means of livelihood has arrived at the most critical period of its history. The existence of the medical doctor is at stake. Competition is becoming sharp, and the effect of this competition is reducing the remuneration of medical men. Many hew healing sects and irregulars have made inroads upon the sum total of patients, originally divided among a few schools. Thus, a score of cults are thriving, partly because they offer the sufferer a new hope, which the old schools have been unable to supply."

75 years later, the same complaint will be made again by orthodox physicians—although it will not appear in print.

1926—

- **Dr. John Lyden**, graduate of American School of Naturopathy, refers to Naturopathy as "Sanipractic", and this term spreads throughout the Pacific Northwest, causing some discord in the naturopathic community. A "Drugless Healers" license had been available since 1919.[*]

- **Lindlahr College of Naturopathy** in Chicago becomes National College of Drugless Physicians, with an expanded curriculum and dual chiropractic and naturopathic programs. R.A. Budden, DM, DC is appointed Dean.

- **John H. Tilden** writes *Toxemia Explained*, a treatise on natural medicine that will enlighten the public and physicians alike to the principles of natural therapeutics.

[*] *Naturopath and Herald of Health*, Aug. 1937, p. 254

- **The Chiropractic-Naturopathic Defense Association** is formed, to combat orthodox medical propaganda and legislation preventing the practice of drugless methods. The organization focuses on the constitutional right of the individual to any type of treatment he desires, they say. Dr. Wolf Adler is president; Dr. Max Warmbrand, vice-president, Dr. Herbert Shelton, treasurer; Dr. Morris March, publicity director, and Mrs. C.B. Schwartz, secretary.

1927—

- **Florida licenses** naturopathic doctors.
- **Oregon also passes** a naturopathic licensing law.

1928—

- **Prosecution of drugless practitioners is stepped up** at the insistence of the orthodox medical profession. In the metropolitan New York area alone, over one hundred chiropractors and naturopaths were charged with practicing medicine without a license in 1928.

- **Emanuel Felke, nature cure pioneer, dies.** The Lutheran pastor who introduced clay applications, iris diagnosis, and complex homeopathic remedies to naturopathic practice, established two sanatariums in Germany. He never charged a fee.

1929—

- **The District of Columbia licenses** naturopathic doctors.

- **U.S. Congress passes legislation recognizing and broadly defining Naturopathy as "any system of healing that does not resort to the use of drugs, [conventional] medicine, or operative surgery for the prevention, relief, or cure of any disease".** It which was signed into law by President Calvin Coolidge.

- A 21-year old **Bernard Jensen** graduates from West Coast Chiropractic College (Oakland, CA) to become the youngest chiropractor in that state. He would then

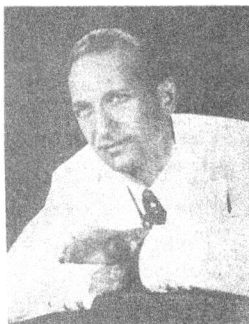

travel east to study at Collins' United States School of Naturopathy and Allied Sciences in New Jersey, becoming one of the DC/ND holders that would be common for the next several decades. Jensen also will study Iridology with Dr. Richard Murell McLain in Oakland and will become over time the foremost exponent of this diagnostic tool in the U.S.

1930—

A surprise testimonial dinner was held to honor Dr. Sinai Gershanek, Dean of the American School of Naturopathy. Students, faculty, and alumni planned the event of June 7th, where nearly two hundred attended. An Article in *Nature's Path* covering the event said "The list of those present was practically a directory of the leaders of Naturopathy and of Chiropractic in the United States and Canada."

Dr. Benedict Lust arrived and joined Dr. and Mrs. Gershanek at the head table, along with Master of Ceremonies Dr. Victor Lindlahr. A vacant seat was adorned with a bowl of red roses to represent the late Louisa Lust.

Dr. Lindlahr, son of the late Henry Lindlahr, had established himself as another of the great American naturopaths with his taking over of his father's practice, as well as teaching and lecturing. He was now promoting the natural health movement with a national lecture series on radio.

Dr. Lindlahr noted that Dr. Gershanek was being lauded for four reasons: It was his fiftieth birthday, it was his thirtieth year as an educator, it was his twentieth wedding anniversary, and it was his fifteenth year as Dean of the American School.

The honorary degree of Doctor of Natural Science was awarded to a number of individuals deemed worthy by the President and Dean. Notable was Dr. Frederick W. Collins, with whom Dr. Gershanek had historically experienced friction. Nevertheless, "in spite of all criss-crossfires and fighting," Dr. Gershanek recognized Dr. Collins, President of First National Naturopathic University ("combining in one a chiropractor, an osteopath, and a naturopath with the skill and techic of all three; [an] author and fighter").

Dr. Teresa M. Shippell, a Director of the ANA and the prime mover in getting Naturopathy recognized by Congress, was honored with the degree.

Next was Dr. W. Robert Keashen, Honorary President of the National Society of Naturopaths and expert biochemist, whose work in researching food chemistry was published in naturopathic journals.

Dr. Clarence R. Rungee, ANA Director in Connecticut; Dr. J. Allerton Choquet, ANA Director in Vermont; Dr. E.W. Cordingly, Indiana ANA Director and editor of *The Naturopathic Bulletin*; and several others were conferred the honorary degree.

Dr. Gershanek referred to Dr. Lust, saying, "In all these years, we have been friends; He has been my patron and benefactor. Those who dared say he is prejudiced and narrow-minded are far, far from the truth. He has made me, *a Jew*--and I am proud of it-- his dean. Is this religious bigotry? Far from it! The clamor and the carping criticisms are now dying a natural death, and out of it all he emerges to remain *our father in Naturopathy*!"

It was reported that "pandemonium and cheers" ensued for ten minutes, "...with all rising and shouting, 'Our Doctor Lust!'"

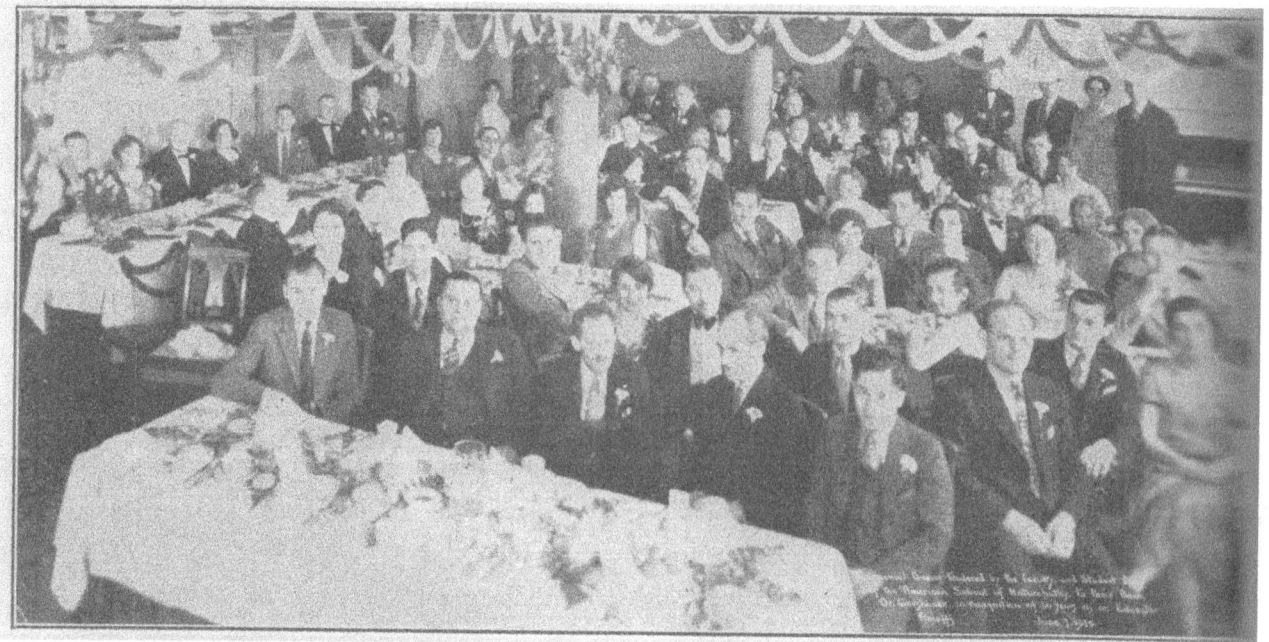

1930—

- **Dr. Frederick W. Collins succeeds in having the New Jersey Supreme Court declare Iridiagnosis to be an exact science.** Dr. Collins was called a "quack" by a Newark medical doctor named Tansey, who stated that iridology was "bunk". Collins sued the man, who produced 22 doctors to testify on his behalf, including Chief Medical Examiner Norris of New York State. On the stand, Dr. Norris was forced to admit that the evidence for the accuracy of diagnosis by the eye indicated that it was in fact a science. Dr. Tansey was directed to pay all court costs, and a considerable sum to Dr. Collins in reparation. Benedict Lust testified in the week-long trial that was reported by the Associated Press. More positive publicity for Naturopathy and another battle won by Dr. Collins.

1931—

- In February, the 70th **US Congress clarified the 1929 Naturopathic Licensing Act** in a second bill. This second bill (HR 12169, "an act to regulate the practice of the healing art to protect the public health in the District of Columbia") amended the 1929 law to approve the practice of naturopathy in the District of Columbia.

Dictionary of Occupational Titles (DOT), the United States Government's book of jobs and job descriptions:

[the naturopathic doctor] Diagnoses, treats, and cares for patients, using a system of practice that bases treatment of physiological functions and abnormal conditions on natural laws governing human body: Utilizes physiological, psychological, and mechanical methods, such as air, water, light, heat, earth, phytotherapy, food and herb therapy, psychotherapy, electrotherapy, physiotherapy, minor and orificial surgery, mechanotherapy, naturopathic corrections and manipulation, and natural methods or modalities, together with natural medicines, natural processed foods and herbs, and nature's remedies. Excludes major surgery, therapeutic use of x-ray and radium, and use of drugs, except those assimilable substances containing elements or compounds of body tissues and are physiologically compatible to body processes for maintenance of life.

- **California Chiropractic College** opens its San Jose campus with its naturopathic program, "incorporating all forms of drugless therapy".

- **The State of Maine licenses naturopaths** in April 1931.

- Benedict Lust's **American School of Naturopathy and Chiropractic moves** to a better location. Its East 35th Street Manhattan facility had been the object of ridicule in a slanderous report published in the Journal of the American Medical Association two years before, to reduce public confidence in Naturopathy. At that time, Lust responded* to the description of the school as a "sorry-looking affair" with the retort, "Bless your venomous heart, we have never seen the day where we would not plead guilty...we have never known anything but poverty in our little 35th Street center where we have kept the torch of nature and reason burning up to the present time."

The new school on East 12th Street is a greatly expanded and enhanced version of the old one, and will accommodate 1000 students. The official dedication will take place in conjunction with the 34th National Convention of the American Naturopathic Association, which will be held this year in the school's new spacious auditorium and classrooms instead of the usual large hotel.

1933—

- The famed **Battle Creek Sanitarium**, the largest natural medicine facility in the world, closes its doors; a victim of the Great Depression. Many of the wealthy who sponsored, supported, and attended "The San" were wiped out in the stock market crash of 1929. It was in vogue for the rich to travel to Michigan to regain their health, but when the economy plunged, fewer could afford it. The less affluent had to make do with their local naturopath.

Meanwhile, elsewhere...
- **Naturopaths in South Africa build a sanatorium** in Johannesburg. Such is its advance publicity that nearly all inpatient rooms are booked even before the facility opens. Next on the agenda for the association is to establish a naturopathic school to be affiliated with the facility.

* "She Stoops to Conquer", *Nature's Path 23:7; pp. 226-239*

SHOW YOUR COLORS

MEDICINE IN THE SKY

M.D.

SUN A·N·A PIN

N.D.

BLUE BLOOD OF RANK

RED BLOOD OF VITALITY

THE PARTING WALL

1934—

- **The University of the Healing Arts** opens in Denver, Colorado. Its natural therapeutics program spreads the work of Tilden.

- **Metropolitan College opens its naturopathic program.** Ernest J. Smith, DM, DC (pictured below), Graduate of National College of Drugless Physicians in Chicago and Western Reserve in Cleveland, founded **Metropolitan College** in Cleveland in 1919.

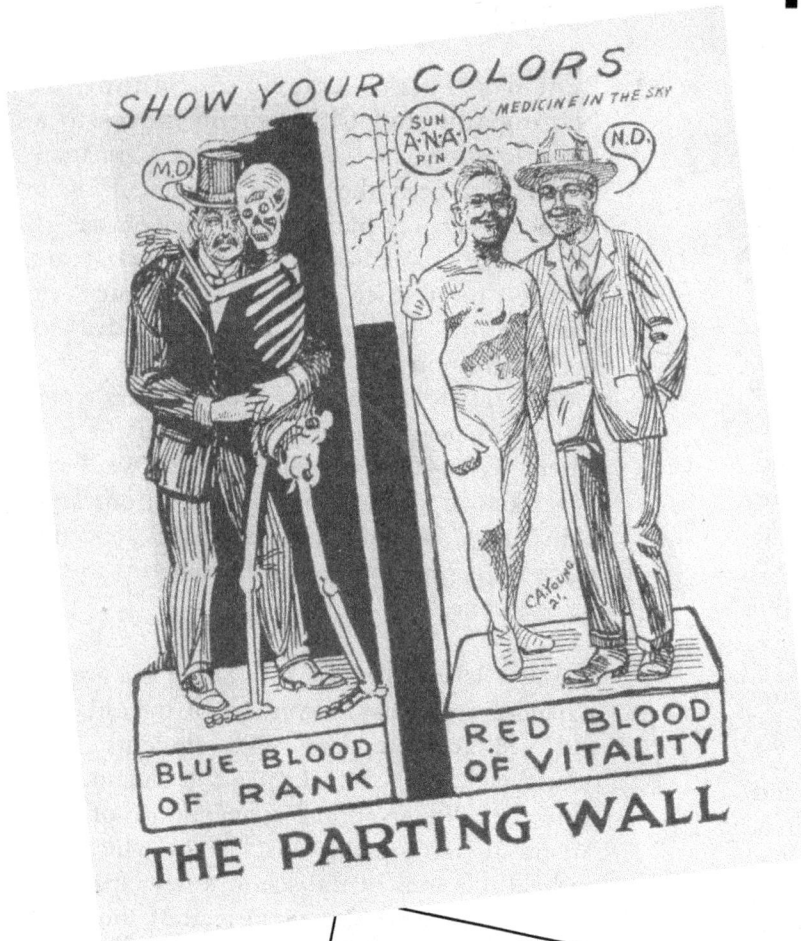

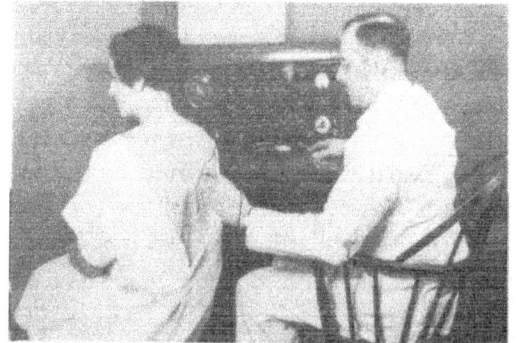

It established one of the first four-year chiropractic programs, at a time when most institutions thought such a lengthy course was economically unfeasible. In 1934 they began conferring their naturopathic degree. Metropolitan was viewed with pride by both naturopathic and chiropractic school associations.

METROPOLITAN COLLEGE CHIROPRACTIC PHYSIOTHERAPY DRUGLESS HEALTH CLINIC MB CLEVELAND, O.

THE METROPOLITAN COLLEGE

INCORPORATED NOT FOR PROFIT

Nationally Recognized and Accredited

TEACHING

CHIROPRACTIC

PHYSIOTHERAPY (Mechanotherapy)

NATUROPATHY

(Member of the International Chiropractic Congress)

Metropolitan College is nationally recognized, and is qualified to teach Chiropractic, Electrotherapy, Mechanotherapy, Naturopathy and other methods of drugless healing. Is authorized by the State of Ohio to confer degrees of Doctor of Chiropractic, Doctor of Electrotherapy and Doctor of Mechanotherapy and Doctor of Naturopathy. The college is located at 3400 Euclid Avenue, Cleveland, Ohio. Established 1919.

CURRICULUM
ORGANIZATION OF DEPARTMENTS

Department of Anatomy

1. Osteology
2. Syndesmology
3. Myology
4. Angiology
5. Splanchnology
   A. Respiratory System
   B. Digestive System
   C. Genito-Urinary System
   D. Ductless Glands
7. Neurology
   A. Brain and Spinal Cord
   B. Spinal and Cranial Nerves
   C. Autonomic Nervous System
8. Special Senses
10. Histology
12. Dissection

Department of Physiology

1. Tissues
4. Blood and Circulation
5. Visceral System
   A. Respiration
   B. Digestion
   C. Secretions and Excretions
6. Metabolism
7. Nervous System
   A. Brain and Spinal Cord
   B. Spinal and Cranial Nerves
   C. Autonomic Nervous System
8. Special Senses

Department of Diagnosis

1. Symptomatology
2. Physical Diagnosis
3. Acute Infectious Diseases
4. Diseases of Blood and Circulation
5. Diseases of Visceral System
   A. Diseases of Respiration
   B. Diseases of Digestion
   C. Diseases of Genito-Urinary System
   D. Diseases of Ductless Glands
6. Diseases of Metabolism
7. Diseases of Nervous System
8. Diseases of Eye, Ear, Nose and Throat
9. Gynecology and Obstetrics

Department of Pathology

1. General and Special Pathology
3. Bacteriology

Department of Chemistry

1. General Chemistry
4. Blood Analysis
5b. Gastric Analysis
5c. Urinalysis

Department of Chiropractic

1. Orthopedy
2. Philosophy
3. Palpation
4. Technique and Drill
5. Abnormalities
7. Soft Tissue Adjusting

Department of Mechano-therapy

1. Basic Principles
2. Food, Fasting, and Mono-Diets
3. Psychotherapy
4. Hydrotherapy
5. Electrotherapy
6. Massage and Manual Therapy
7. Posture and Corrective Exercises
8. Foot Correction
9. Light Therapy
10. Dermatomes
11. Vaso-Motor Control of Circulation
12. Colonic Irrigation
13. First Aid and Minor Surgery

Department of Naturopathy
includes

Phytotherapy   Hygiene
Dietetics   First Aid
Electrotherapy   Sanitation
Mechanotherapy   Heliotherapy

Special Subjects

1. Terminology
2. Hygiene
4. First Aid
5. Dietetics
6. Roentgenology
7. Jurisprudence

The Staff reserves the right to augment or alter the curriculum as necessary to improve scholastic standards.

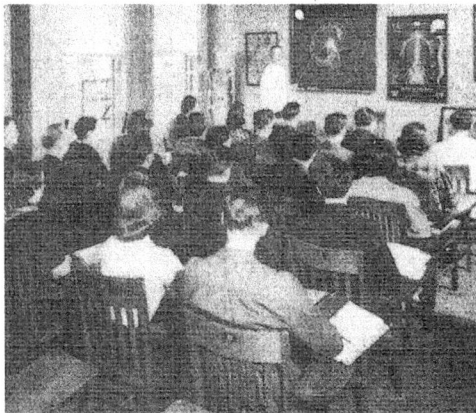

Pathology class

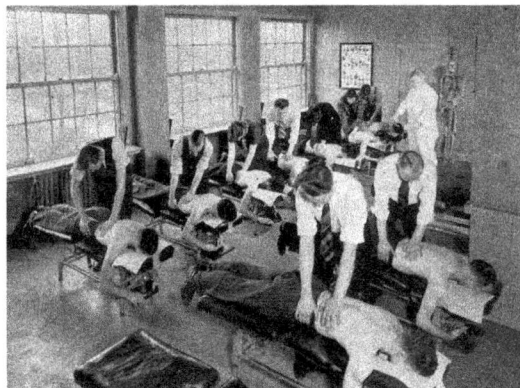

Spinal manipulation was taught in all programs. Here, the students are practicing the Collins Universal Naturopathic Technique, as originated by Frederick Collins at the First National University in New Jersey.

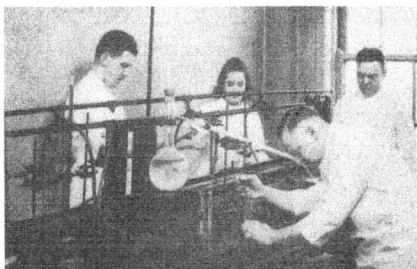

Chemistry class at Metropolitan

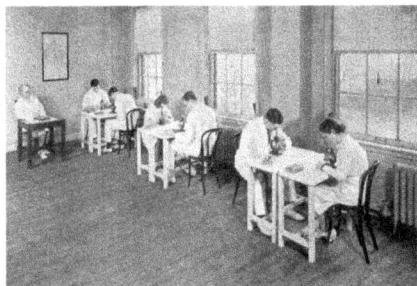

Basic microbiology was required for NDs

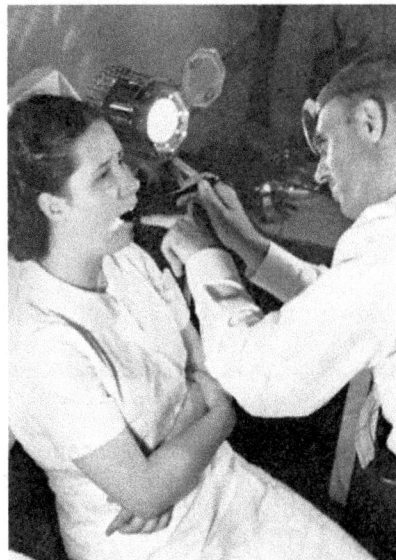

Otolaryngology training enabled the progressive ND to take care of many common complaints

31

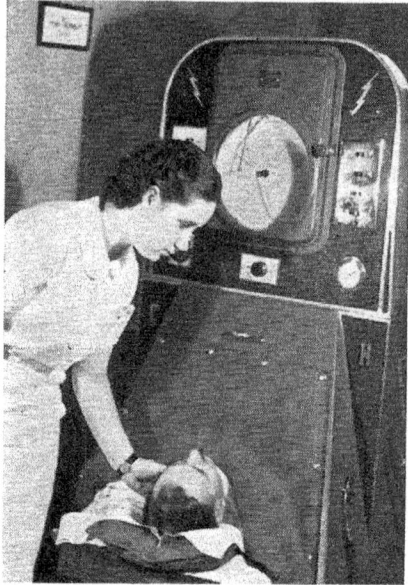

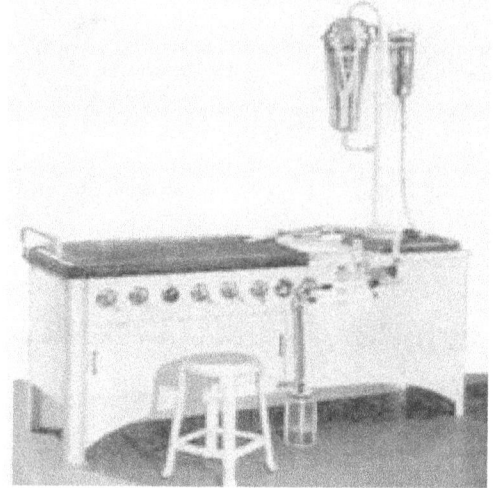

Hyperthermia therapy was used extensively in the Metropolitan clinic, and this fundamental nature cure method used up-to-date technology to achieve its effects.

Colonic irrigation, a form of internal hydrotherapy, is a powerful tool for detoxification. With temperature- and pressure-controlled water clearing the contents of the colon, the "colonic" was a mainstay in naturopathic clinics.

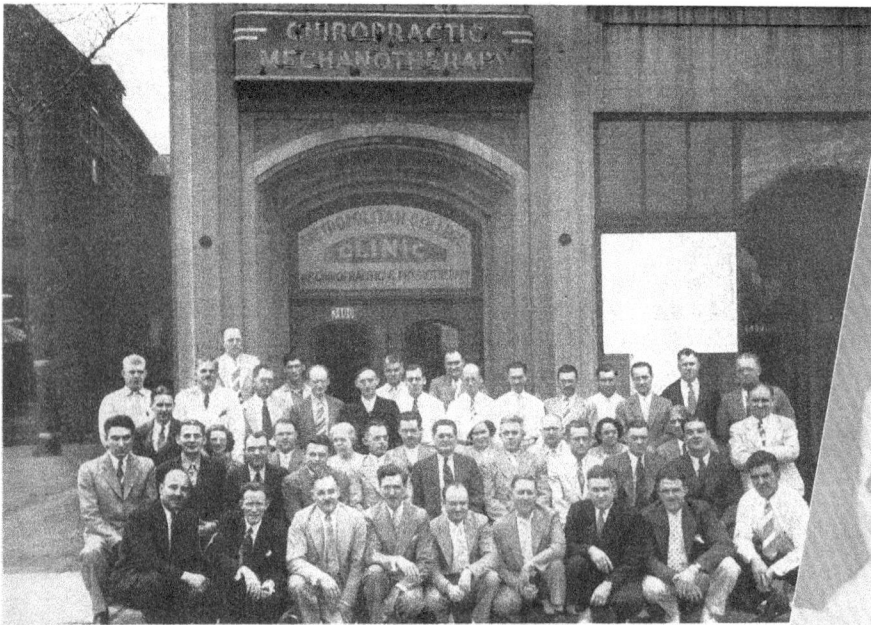

POST-GRADUATE CLASS IN NATUROPATHY.

A class of NDs at Metropolitan. Mechanotherapy was licensed in Ohio, but Naturopathy was not (which explains its absence on the sign in the photo). Those students native to Ohio typically took the mechanotherapy program because the curriculum was substantially the same as the naturopathic program and they could be licensed.

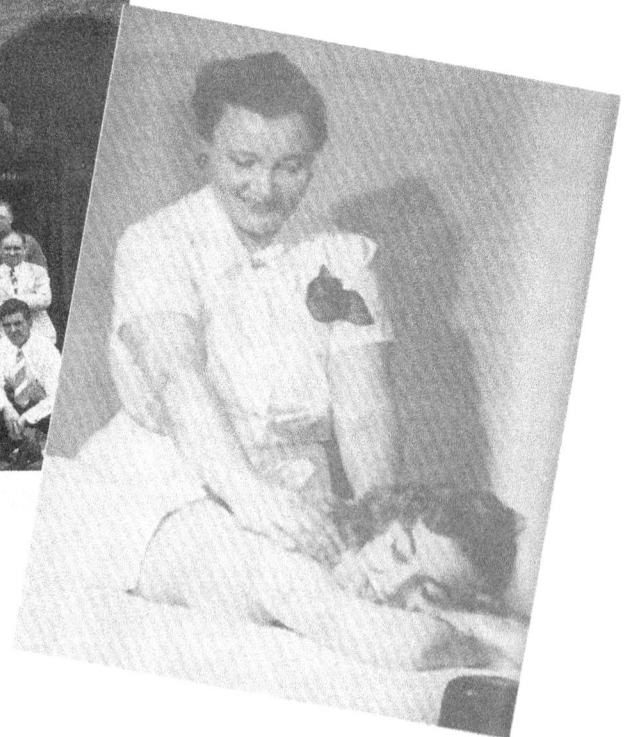

Massage therapy has been a modality in natural therapeutics since the beginning.

GADGETS! While the fundamentalist *Natural Hygiene* movement continued to use only fasting and dietary regulation to effect their cures, the mainstream ND took the traditional applications of water and manipulations to a higher level. More powerful uses of natural agents such as water, heat, cold, light, and mechanical manipulations could be used to get better results faster. The American Naturopathic Association approved these advancements, noting that they augmented *"nature's agencies and forces"*, as described in most legal definitions of Naturopathy.

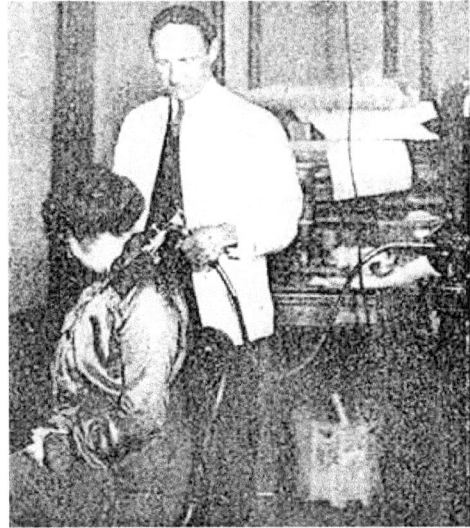

Joe Shelby Riley, DC, ND applies a mechanical concussor to the spine of a patient at National University of Therapeutics in Washington, D.C. Riley was one of the "Big Five" naturopathic pioneers.

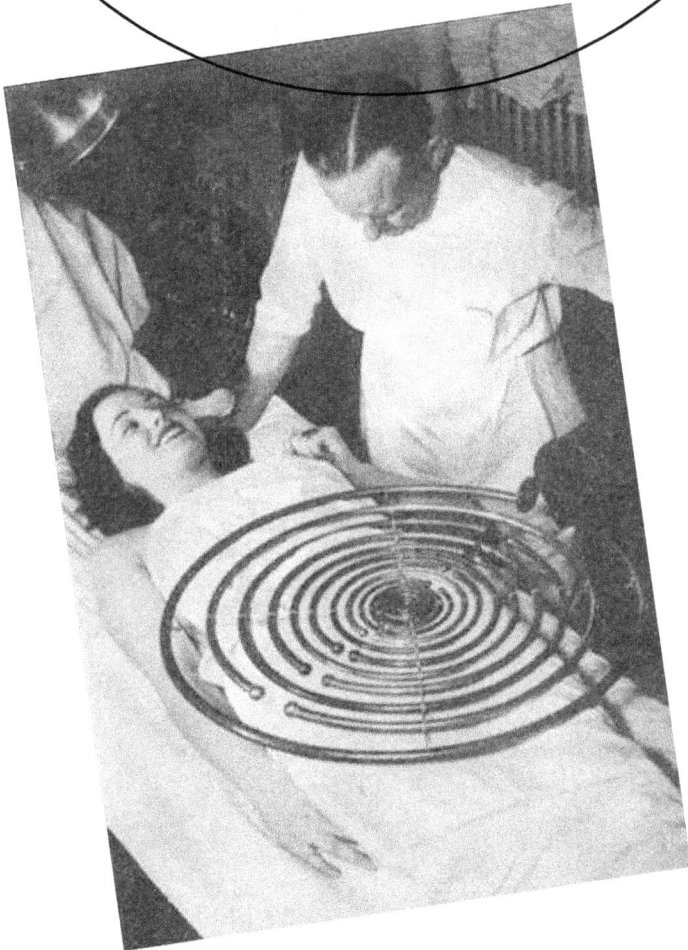

A multiple wave oscillator is placed over the patient to use high frequency electrical energy to revitalize cells.

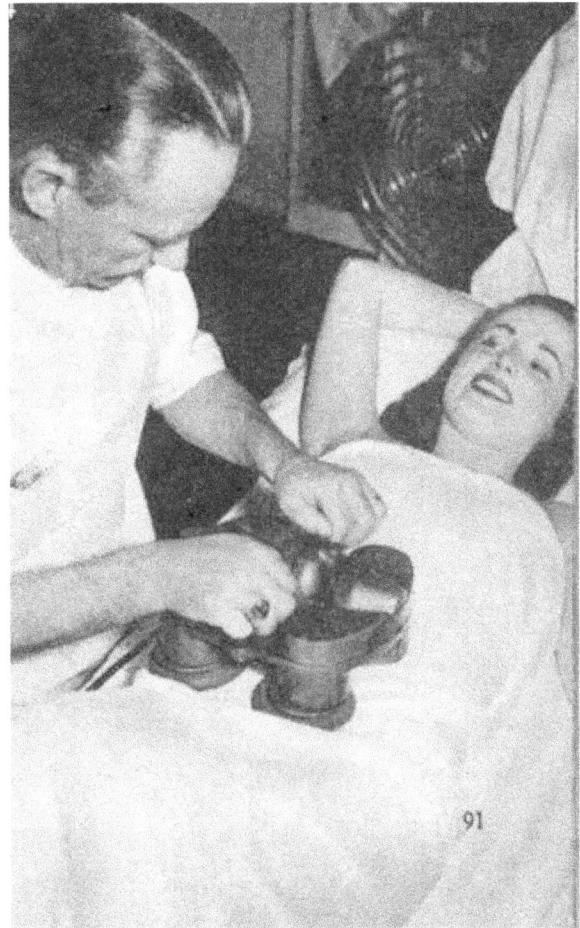

Why use your hands to laboriously massage the abdomen when the internal organs can benefit from *thousands* of impulses in the same length of time?

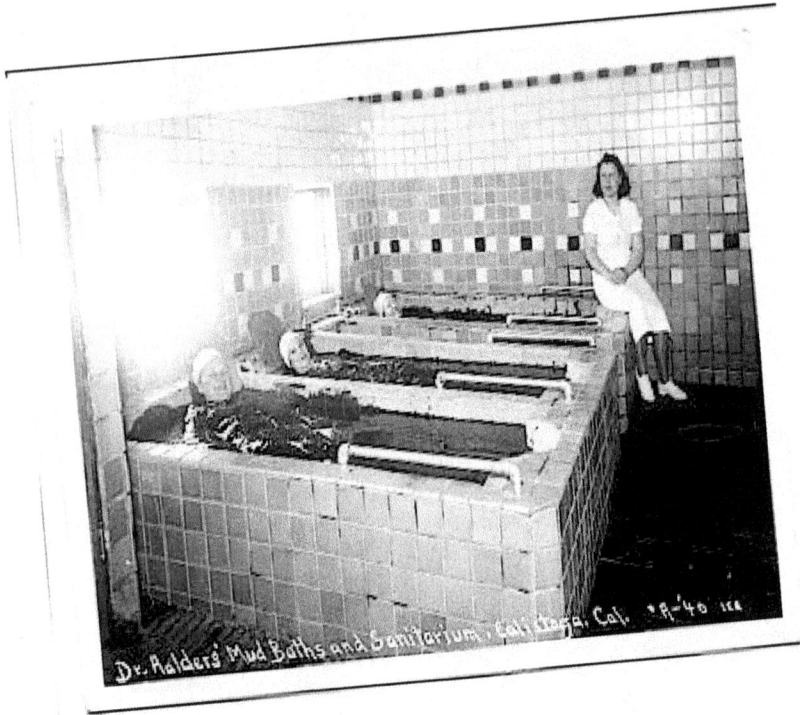

Healing clay in the form of mud baths, applied in a Calistoga, California sanatorium of a Dr. Aalder.

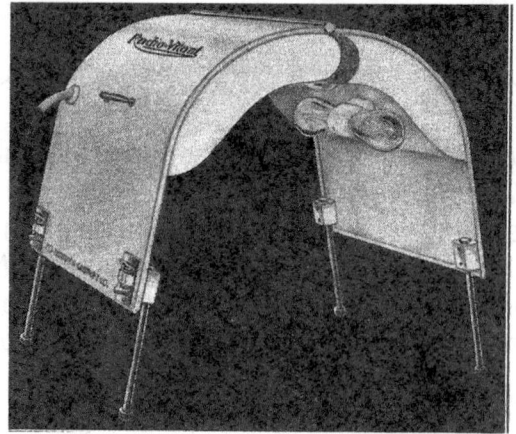

A cradle baker, for applying radiant heat to the body.

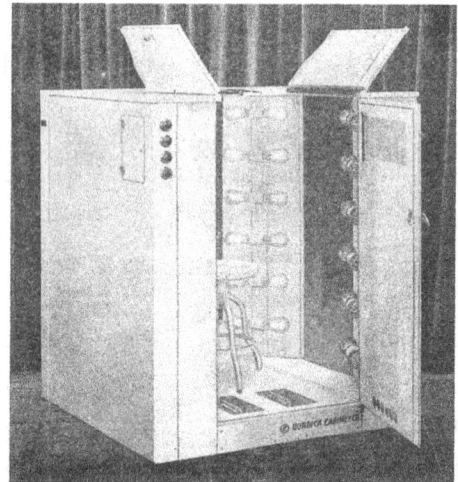

The light cabinet was once a common fixture in natural therapy offices.

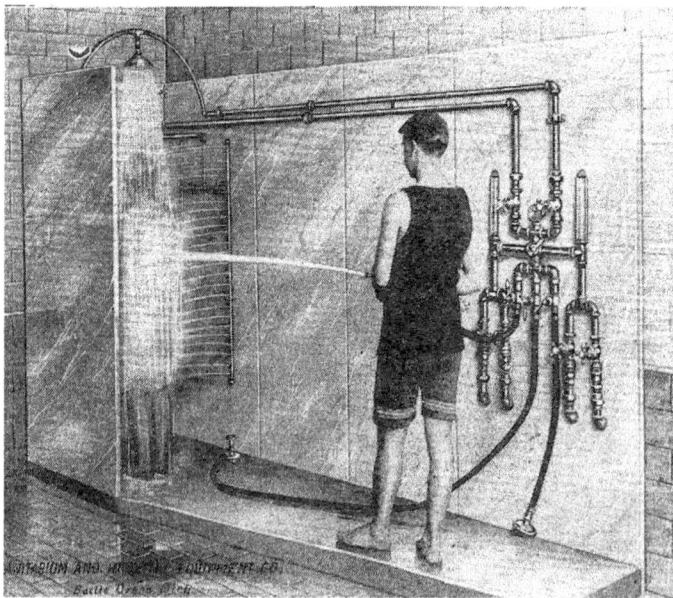

The Scotch douche, a hydrotherapy mainstay, as made famous at the Battle Creek Sanitarium.

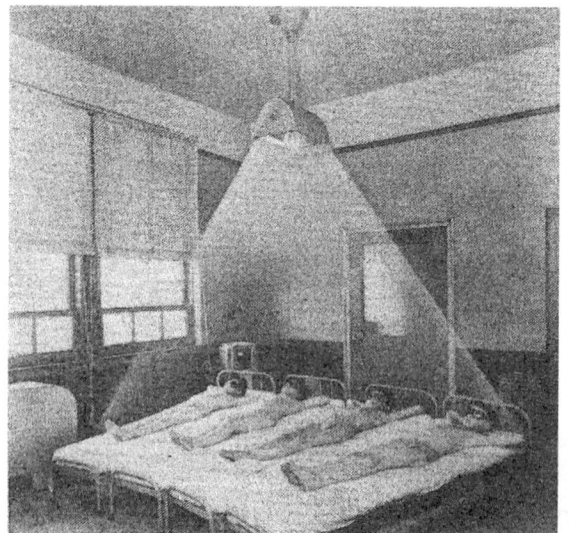

Artificial sunlight could be concentrated and used to treat several persons at once.

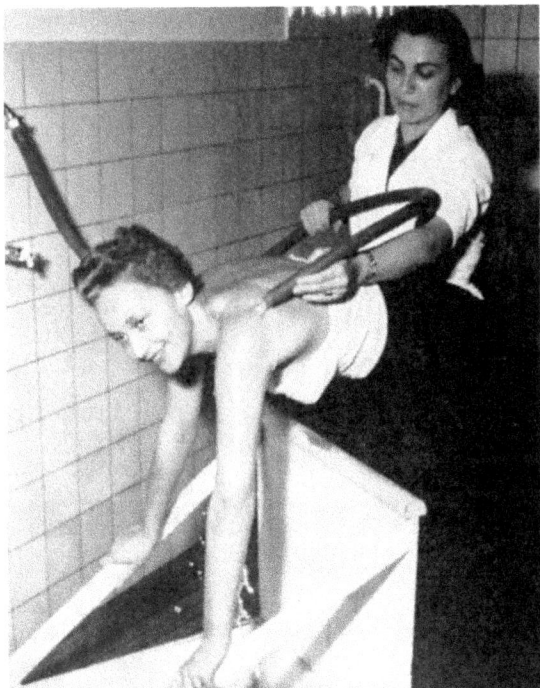

The hydrotherapy maneuver known as the "arm gush".

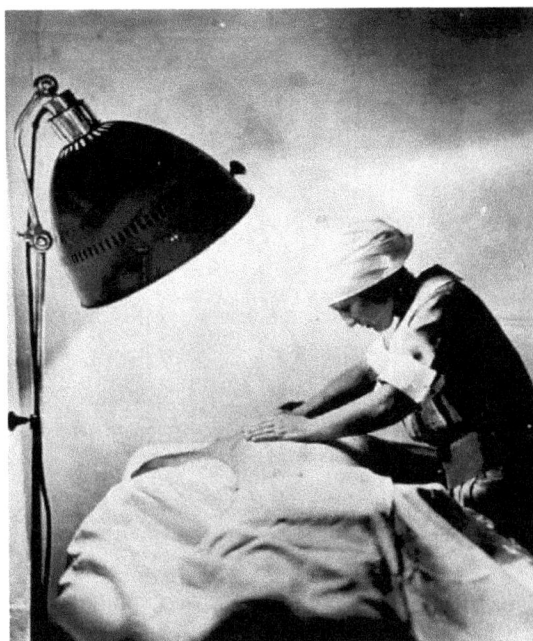

Infrared light coupled with soft tissue manipulation.

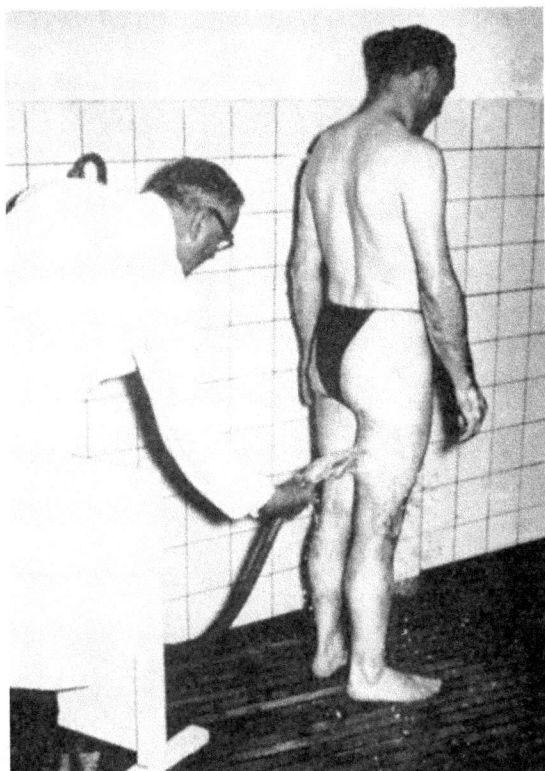

The "Leg gush".

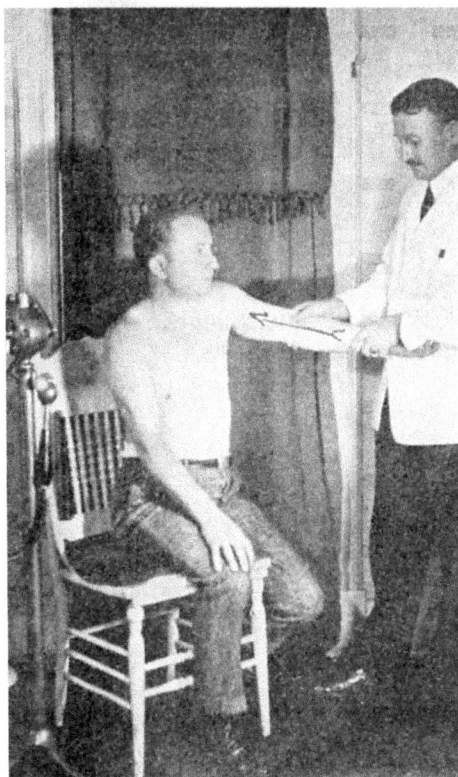

Peter Puderbach, ND demonstrates extremity soft tissue manipulation.

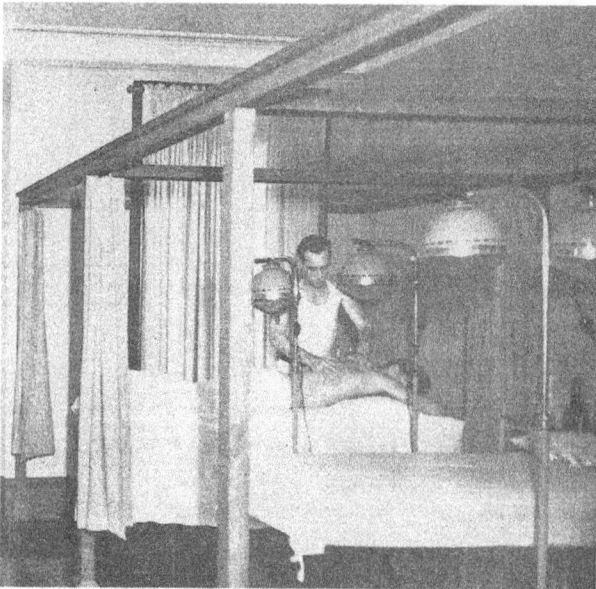

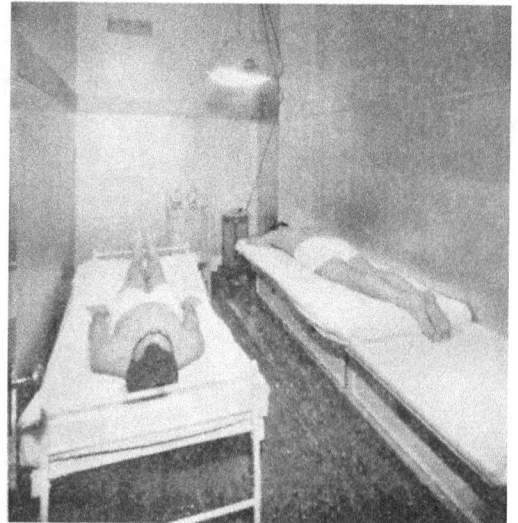

More ultraviolet therapy in Dr. Resnick's facility.

Once again, infrared and massage are combined at the Kenmore Health Club in Boston.

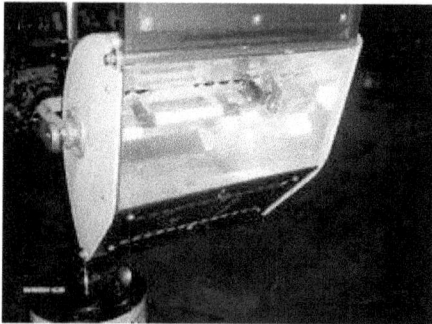

A close-up look at a hot quartz ultraviolet lamp, capable of delivering many health benefits.

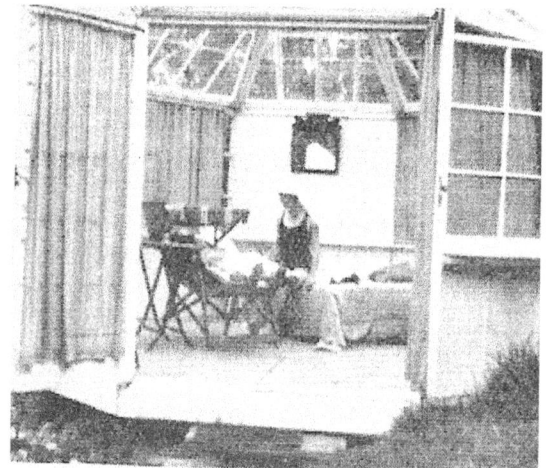

A unique heliotherapy setup: a revolving chalet made of "vitaglass"—quartz glass that allows all the sun's rays to penetrate. The platform rotates to follow the sun and allows a controlled environment for the patient to absorb as much of the rays as possible without effort.

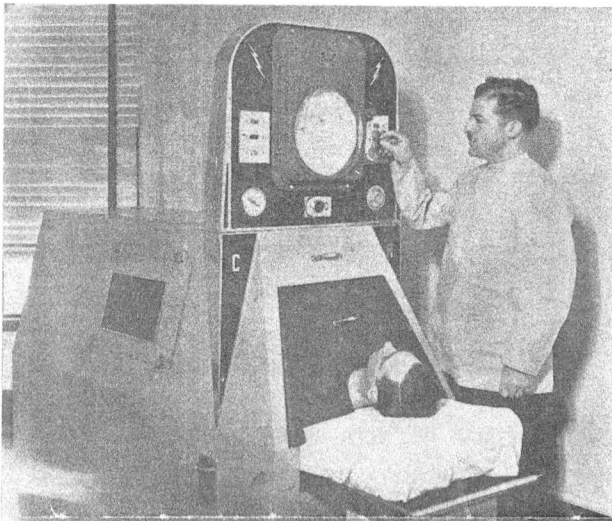

Dr. Sarle Resnick adjusts the controls on his fever cabinet. Slowly heating the body under controlled conditions creates the healing response essential to "nature cure".

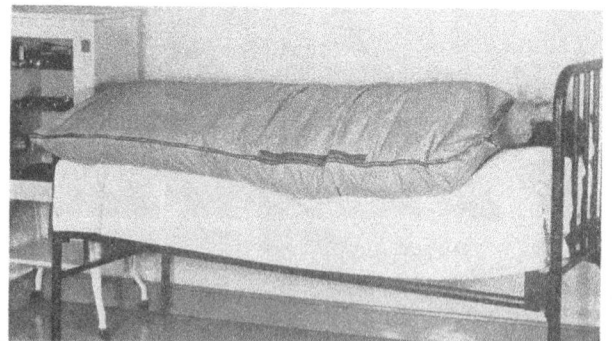

A less complicated device for hyperpyrexia: a sleeping bag with hot air pumped into it.

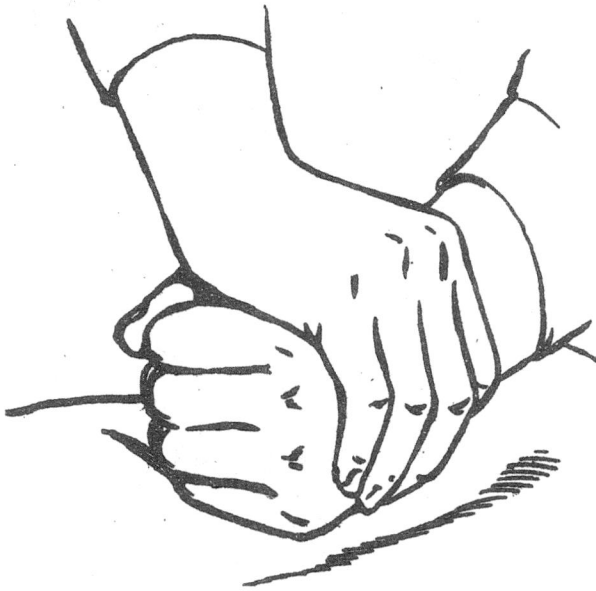

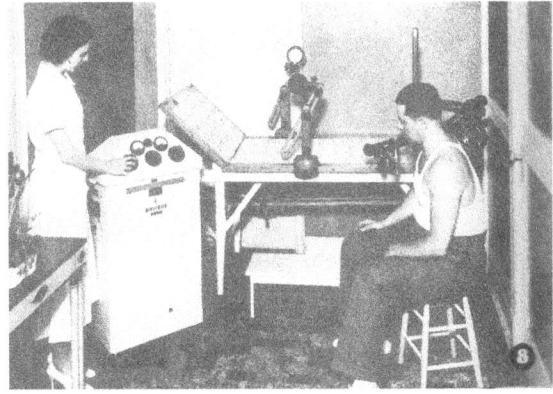

Short wave diathermy applied to an injured shoulder, in a facility also offering hydrotherapy, massage, light therapy, and other modalities.

Manipulation of the joints has been part of naturopathic methodology since the early days. This illustration from a textbook points up the fact that chiropractic, osteopathic, and naturopathic methods often overlap, depending on the original influence in the particular school the ND attended. Nevertheless, some original techniques developed that do not appear in any chiropractic or osteopathic curriculum.

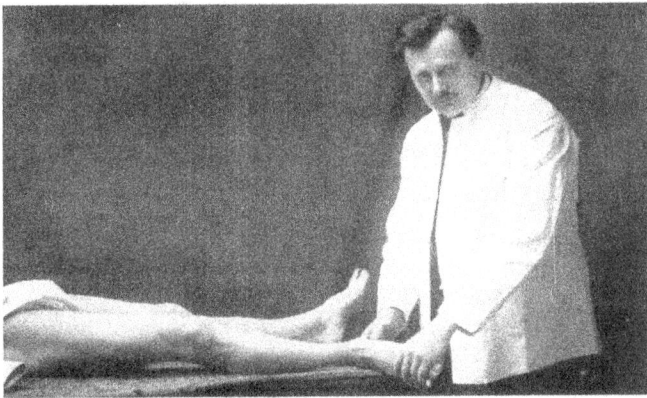

Intermittent motorized traction.

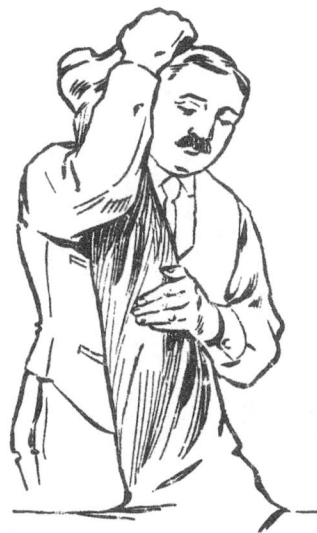

Dr. Frederick Collins, a master of physical methods and manipulation, demonstrates a maneuver.

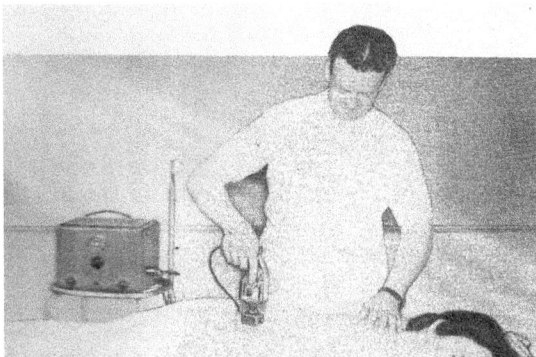

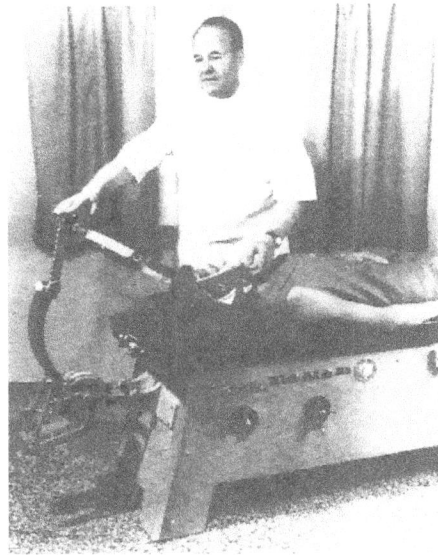

A device using sound waves to change the tone of the spinal muscles and ligaments.

Part of a naturopathic protocol for treating sciatica.

37

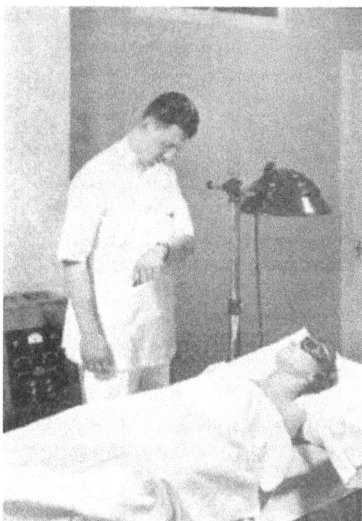

Often, naturopathic doctors had their offices in their homes. They continued to, even after medical doctors discontinued the practice. Patients who preferred natural treatment also preferred the cozy environment.

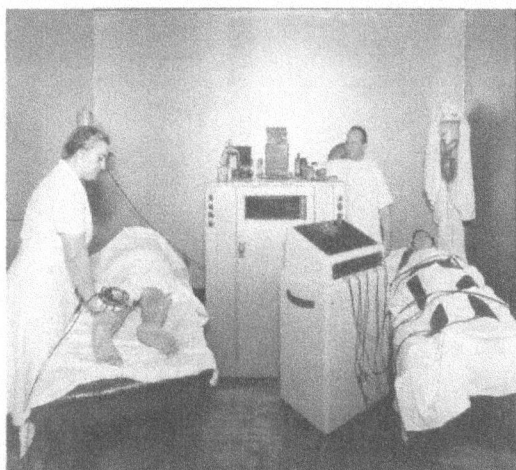

Electrotherapy and massage being applied. Colonic irrigation device is at the ready in the back of the room.

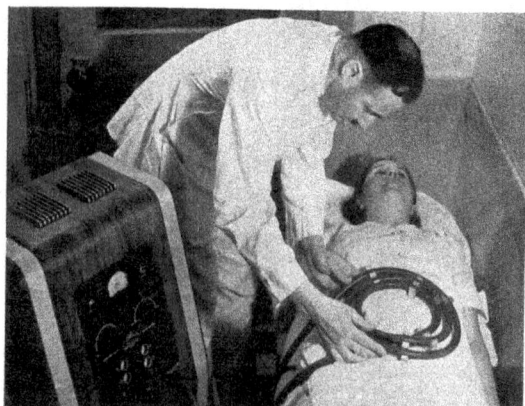

A "pancake coil" is applied to a patient receiving short wave treatment. The heat induced by the machine increases circulation and detoxification in the abdominal organs.

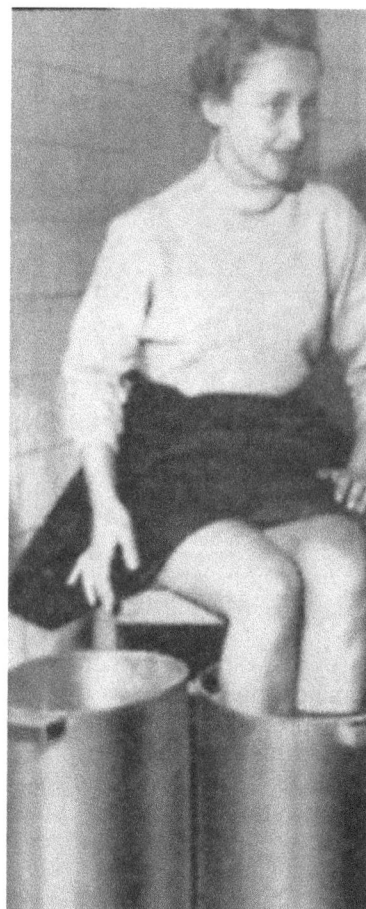

Extremity contrast hydrotherapy. The legs are moved from hot water to cold and back again, to rejuvenate valvular action in the veins.

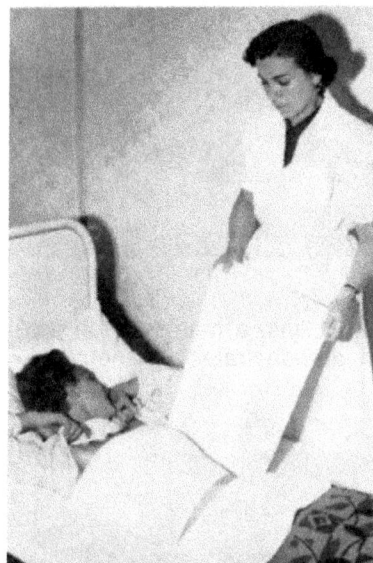

Constitutional hydrotherapy, a form of contrast thermal effects, uses hot and cold towels to stimulate a healing response. A variation on older methods, this method was developed by Otis G. Carroll, ND, of Spokane. It combined hydrotherapy with spinal electrotherapy, a unique approach at the time.

38

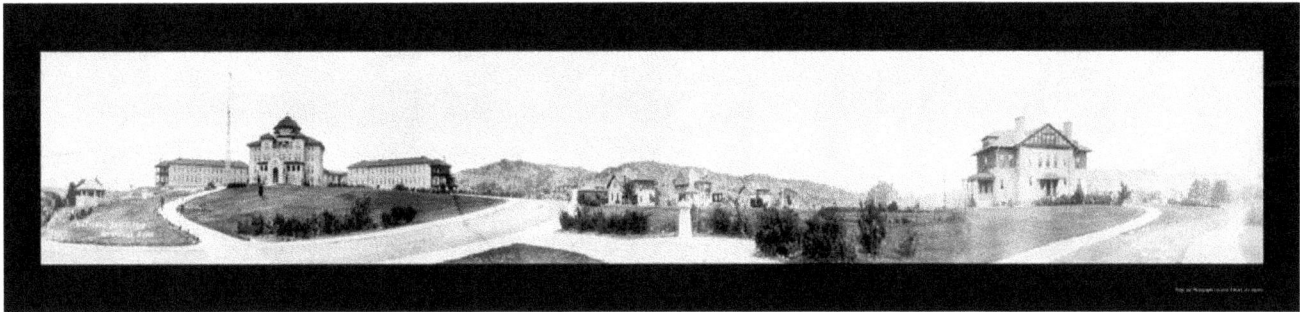

National Sanitarium, Hot Springs, Arkansas. America soon had her own tradition of healing waters, no different than that of Europe.

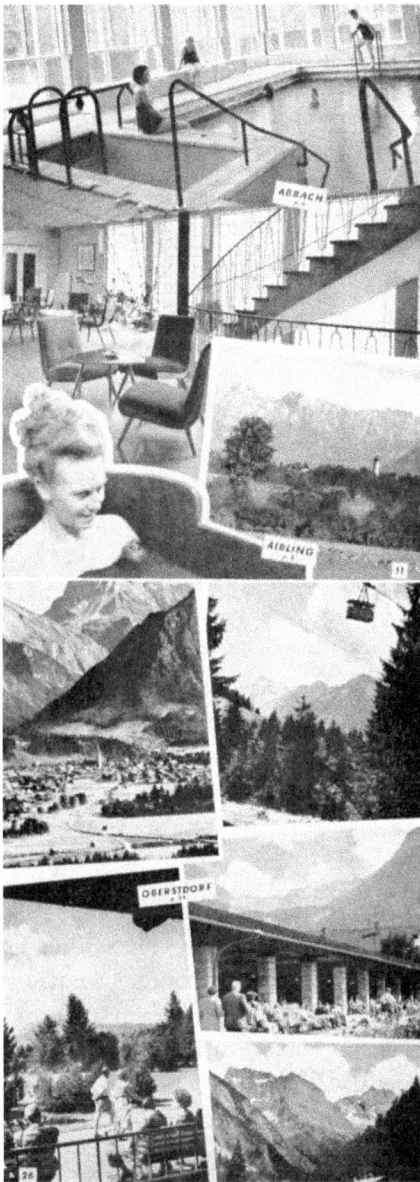

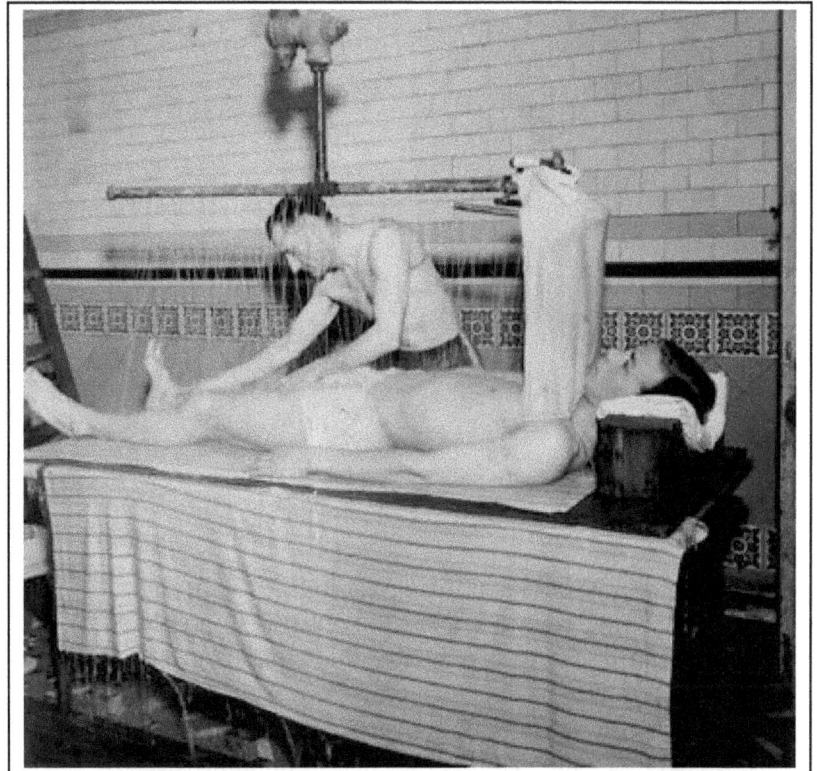

Above: "Vichy douche" hydrotherapy and massage combined. Low-tech, but powerful enough to have an effect on serious disease.

Snapshots of the various nature cure facilities in the Alps, where it all came from.

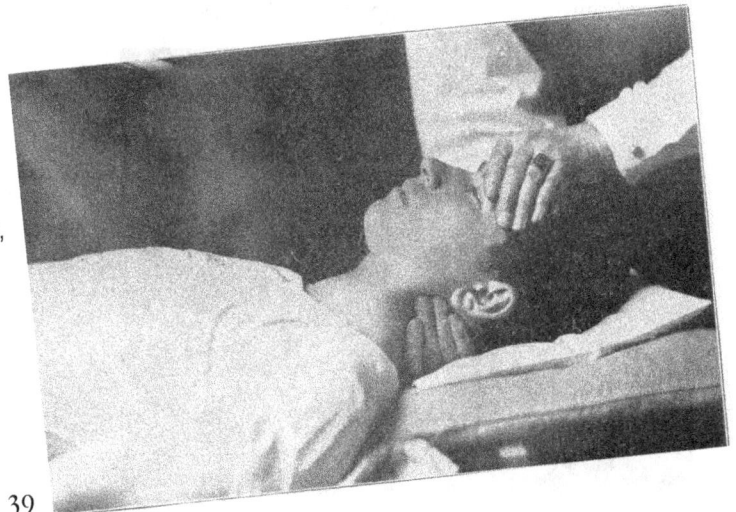

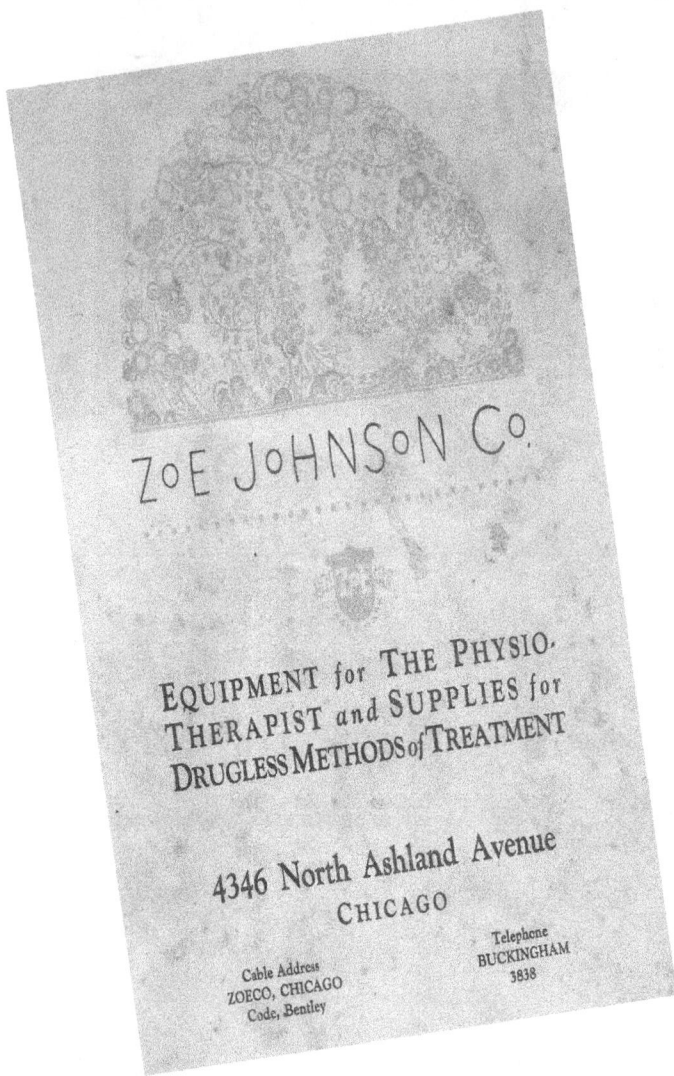

ZOE JOHNSON CO.

EQUIPMENT for THE PHYSIO-
THERAPIST and SUPPLIES for
DRUGLESS METHODS of TREATMENT

4346 North Ashland Avenue
CHICAGO

Cable Address
ZOECO, CHICAGO
Code, Bentley

Telephone
BUCKINGHAM
3838

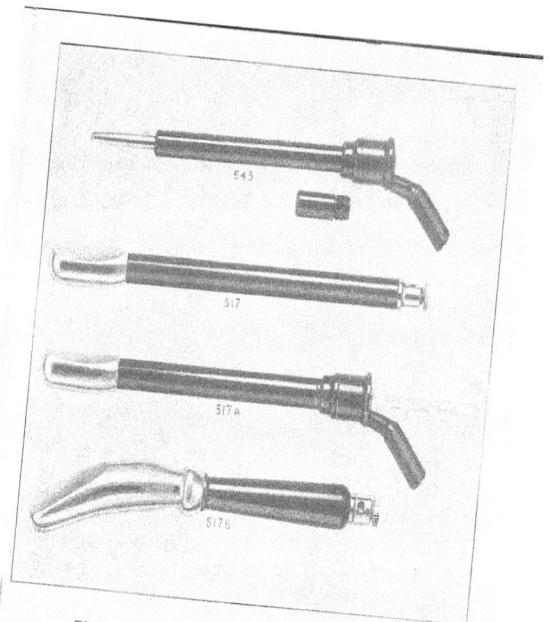

PROSTATIC & VAGINAL ELECTRODES
Constructed with hard rubber shanks and highly polished metal ends,
correctly curved.

Catalog No.		Price
517	Prostatic Electrode	$3.75
517 A	Prostatic Electrode	10.00
517 B	Simpson combination Prostatic and Vaginal Electrode	6.00
343	Corbus Thermaphore (with thermometer arrangement and two insulators). The nickel silver shell measures 5 mm. in diameter. The longer insulator measures 12 cm. and the shorter 2.1 cm. in length, permitting an extension of the electrode to 13 cm. and 4 cm. respectively. Suitable for use in the female cervical and urethral canal, and also in the male urethral canal. A thermometer (not illustrated) may be inserted to the full depth of the electrode, and a reading taken from the exposed end, which is graduated. This electrode is widely used in the treatment of genito-urinary diseases of both sexes.	10.00

Those who used spinal manipulation (as did most naturopaths) needed good treatment tables. Hydrotherapy required containers and equipment also; the various forms of electrotherapy that were bringing drugless methods into the modern age had a number of machines, and almost as many manufacturers. When looking over the equipment suppliers of the period, it is evident that the naturopaths were the practitioners that the public and the vendors alike associated with physical therapies of all types.

While conventional physicians increasingly used the various forms of electrotherapy also, the drugless practitioner embraced these methods because it gave them a more rapid way to reverse conditions characterized by tissue changes (dysplasia, hyperplasia, etc.) and procedures they could apply in acute conditions. Ironically, many of these methods that were used with outstanding success by both camps are now relegated to the "ancient quackery" category. Orthodox medicine found that drugs and surgery was an easier and more profitable way to treat many conditions than electrotherapy; modern naturopaths at the end of the 20th Century would be loathe to return to any methods that were abandoned by the medical establishment for fear of looking like charlatans.

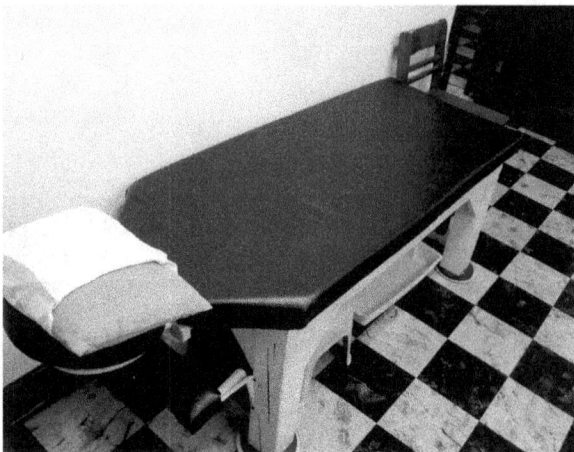

against attempts by the medical establishment to close them down. They were repeatedly successful. The fascinating Spears story is told in the hard-to-find book, *The Lengthening Shadow*. Spears Hospital included many natural therapeutics besides chiropractic manipulation.

The Alta Vista Hospital of Los Angeles became a target for vested interests to limit access to natural

therapies for serious diseases. It would be raided on spurious charges in order to interfere with its operations.

Dr. Benedict Lust followed up the success of his New Jersey "Yungborn" health retreat with one in Florida.

Leo Spears, DC single-handedly established the first chiropractic hospital in Denver, Colorado. Like Benedict Lust, he and his heirs had to constantly fight

After Shelton, William Esser was probably the best-known exponent of Natural Hygiene. He fasted thousands of patients.

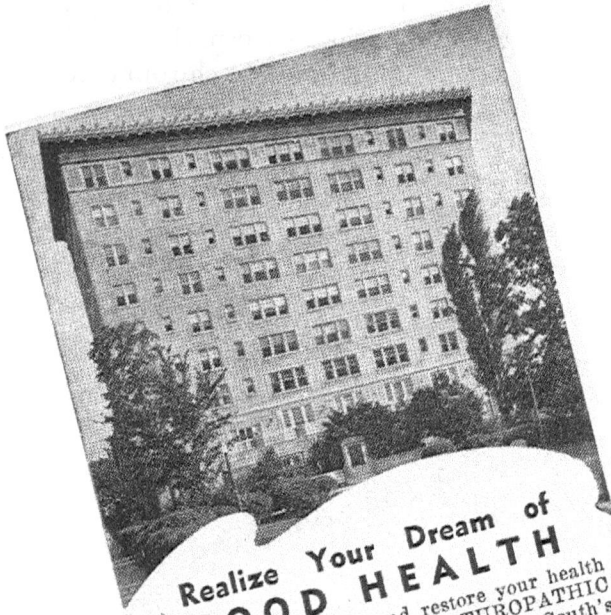

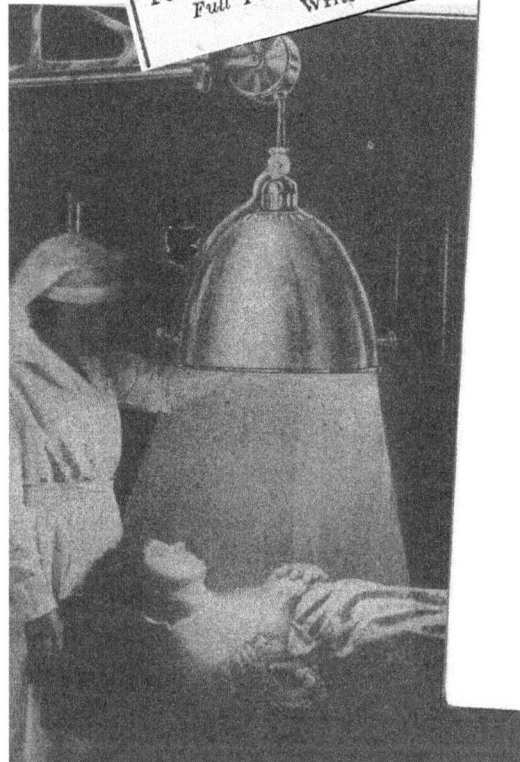

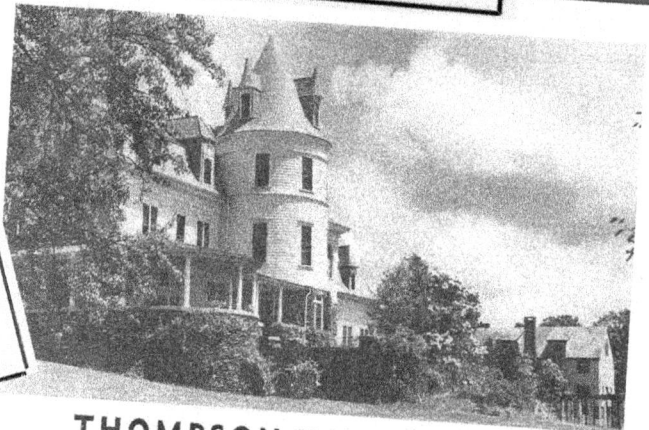

42

The orthodox medical profession took notice of thousands of health care dollars finding their way into other pockets. While efforts were made to discredit the "irregular" practitioners and legislative efforts were made to prevent them from being licensed, another strategy began to be employed. If the public wanted these therapies so badly, they said, *we* will provide them. Thus began a publicity campaign to convince the public that the only really *safe* place for these methods was in the hands of an MD.

This advertisement from *Life* Magazine shows the extent to which this was employed. It tells the reader they will see this kind of diathermy equipment "only in hospitals and doctors' offices. That's where it belongs because that's where it will be properly used."

One will notice that some establishments (such as Esser's Sanatorium) simply used fasting and dietary adjustment, while others used a full range of therapies to restore the sick to health. It must be borne in mind that this was not a feature of only the large facilities. Most individual practitioners of this time were using a variety of methods within the broad definition of Naturopathy. The DC/ND practitioners, who were numerous, of course used spinal manipulation as a major tool. But if they had ND after their names, it was likely that they were *mixers*—a term used within the Chiropractic community to designate one who used therapies other than manipulation. But while most who consulted such doctors did so initially for a muscular problem, they soon found that those therapies being used were also having an effect on organic disease. Soon, many people were considering their naturopath to be their family doctor. Seeing an MD was a last resort.

On a final note, the ad warns: "In all medical matters, rely on your doctor!" (with an emphatic exclamation point).

At this point in time, most *physiotherapy*— infra-red, ultraviolet, diathermy, electrotherapy, muscular re-education, mechanical percussion, hydrotherapy, etc. —was being performed by Doctors of Naturopathy, Doctors of Chiropractic, or Doctors of Mechanotherapy. The separately-licensed field of Physical Therapy had not yet been established.

The orthodox medical profession took notice of thousands of health care dollars finding their way into other pockets.

Joe Shelby Riley, ND, would address the convention of the American Naturopathic Association the next year [in 1935], pointing out that for years the American Medical Association opposed physiotherapy (or Physical Therapy, as it would become more popularly known), which was being administered by naturopaths, chiropractors, and other drugless healers. Then, in an issue[*] of the Journal of the American Medical Association, the AMA reversed their stance:

"The committee previously suggested that physical therapy be considered as an adjunct to other forms of treatment, both medical and surgical. The committee now wishes to suggest that, whereas physical therapy is a smaller and less developed field than either medicine or surgery, and whereas frequently the use of physical measures is merely an adjunct to the other forms of treatment, it is possible to conceive of instances in which the use of some physical measure will be the primary method of treatment, and medical agents and surgical procedures will be the adjunct."

Dr. Riley said, "With great elaboration they describe and mention these physical therapy agents by name. Among these they mention heat, massage, hydro-therapy, infra-red generators, diathermy, electricity, etc. They are incorporating these things into their own work, and will deny them to the drugless profession. Will you let them do it?
...This same battle is raging in the District of Columbia, where the common enemy has made heavy appropriations to put all drugless cults out of business, as well as the Eclectic and Homeopathic schools of medicine. "

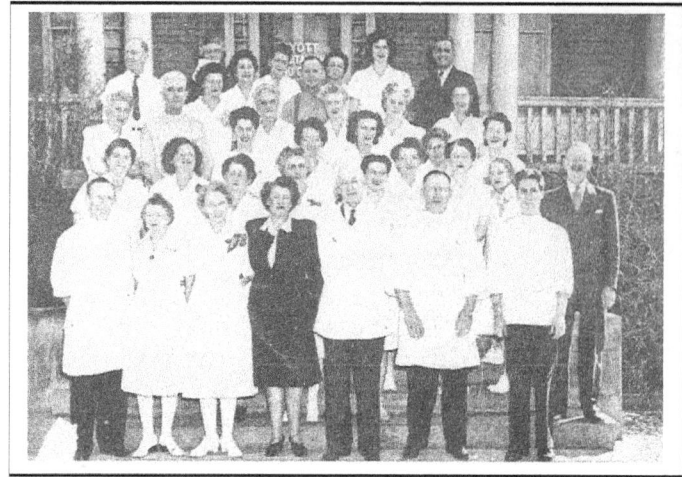

The Pyott Sanitarium in Salt Lake City, Utah was a model for naturopathic clinics everywhere. W.H. Pyott, DC, ND stands in the middle of the front row. With an impressive staff and an even more impressive array of therapies, the Pyott Sanitarium garnered a solid reputation for curing hopeless cases. Pyott would later donate the facility to the profession, and it would become the American Naturopathic Hospital, where NDs across the country could send their difficult cases.

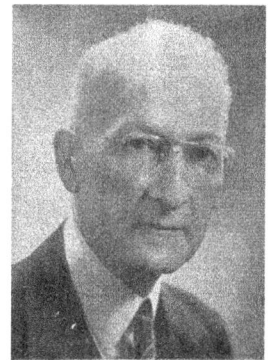

W.H. Pyott, ND

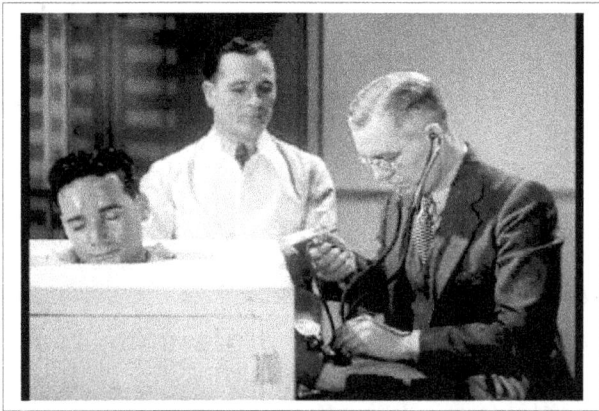

"Anti-quackery" short films were used by the conventional medical community to dissuade people from having their life savings (and their lives!) stolen by phony doctors like naturopaths. In the excerpt above, the unfortunate victim is being cooked in a cabinet that—of course!—has no benefit.

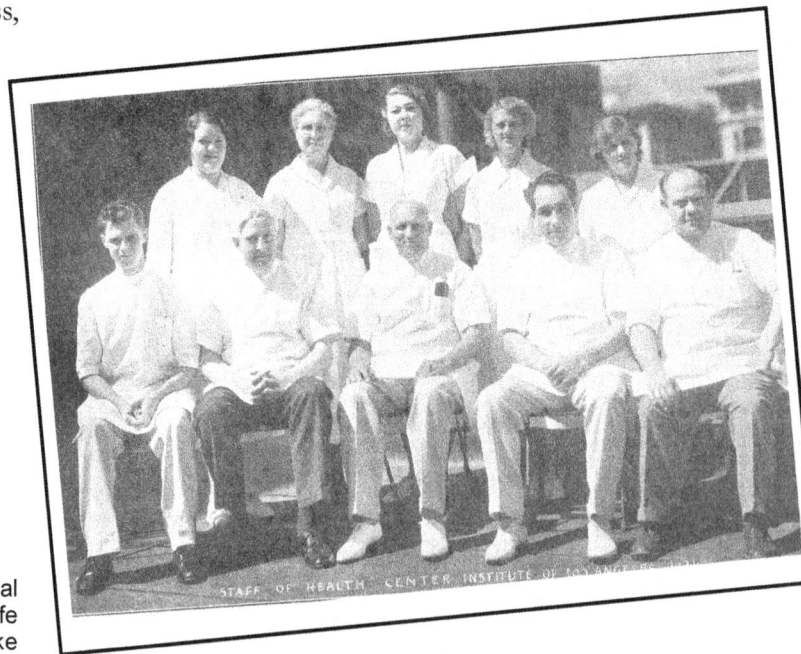

Health Center Institute, Los Angeles

[*] JAMA Aug 27, 1935; p. 585

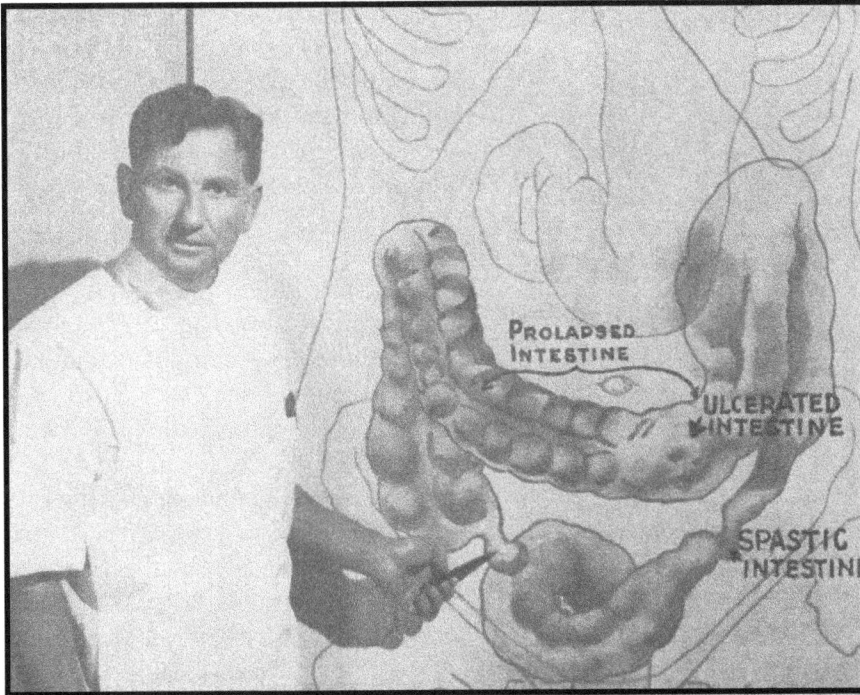

Paul Bragg, ND. Given up to die from tuberculosis as a teenager, he traveled to Switzerland, where he was cured with natural therapeutics administered by the famous Dr. August Rollier. This set his life's path, and Bragg would later restore to health such luminaries as J.C. Penney, Conrad Hilton, and Dr. Scholl (of Dr. Scholl's foot care products). He became famous in the Hollywood and filmmaking community because of his celebrity patients. Finding this an effective way to spread the word about natural medicine, he became what was probably the first "media doctor" in the natural medicine profession. Because of his frequent lectures, he attracted and mentored many who would go on to become famous in their own rights. Jack LaLanne, the exercise and health guru who would use television to preach the value of natural health, was detoxified by Bragg as a young man. V.E. Irons was similarly saved from invalidism and an early death by Bragg. Irons went on to found one of the first all-natural vitamin companies and was a founder of the National Health Federation.

Bragg's name is still on the label of several quality health products he originated, even today. He operated the first known health food store in the country, and is credited with introducing pineapple juice to the American diet. He is rightly called the "Father of the Health Food Movement" in the U.S. His contribution to the acceptance of naturopathic principles by the public is beyond estimation, yet he is largely ignored in the history of the profession.

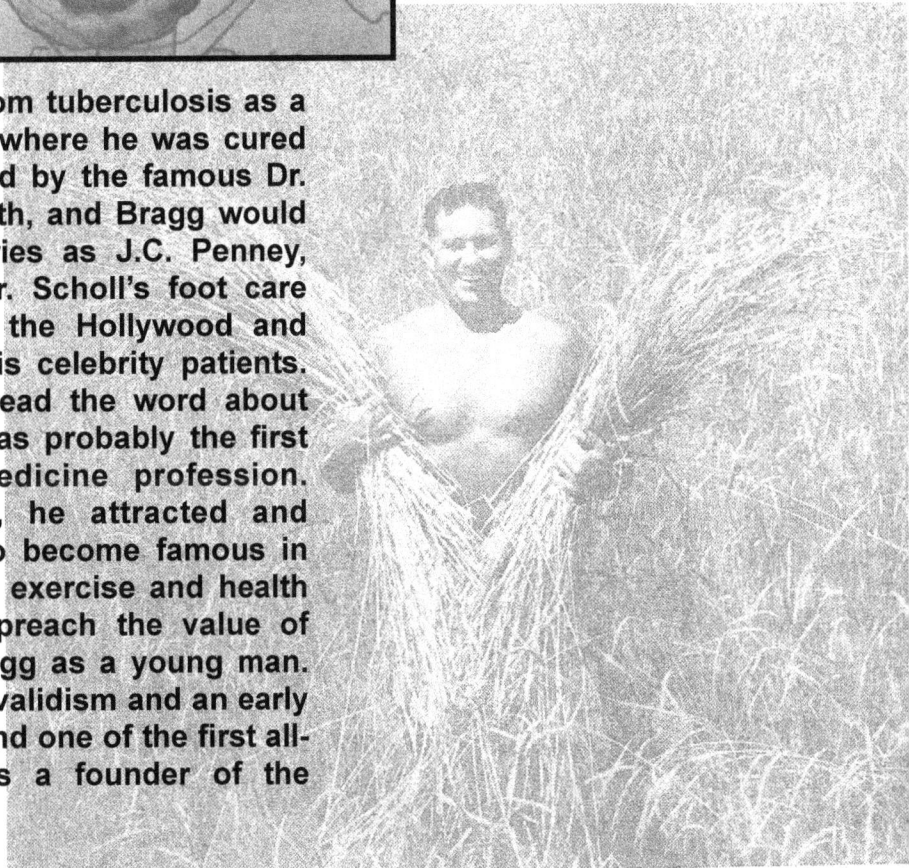

Bragg with the grain to which he attributed his stamina. Four times a week, he ate "Bragg Meal"-- a mixture of rye, barley, oats, wheat, rice bran, and wheat germ that had been *dextrinized*, converting the starch into invert sugar, "the source of all energy".

45

Yet, for all the refinement and proliferation of the field, despite licensing laws being enacted in many states, there was rarely a rest from the opposition. The medical lobby in every state that licensed naturopaths was dedicated to eliminating the profession. It didn't seem to matter whether you were practicing with or without a license—sooner or later, trouble came to your door.

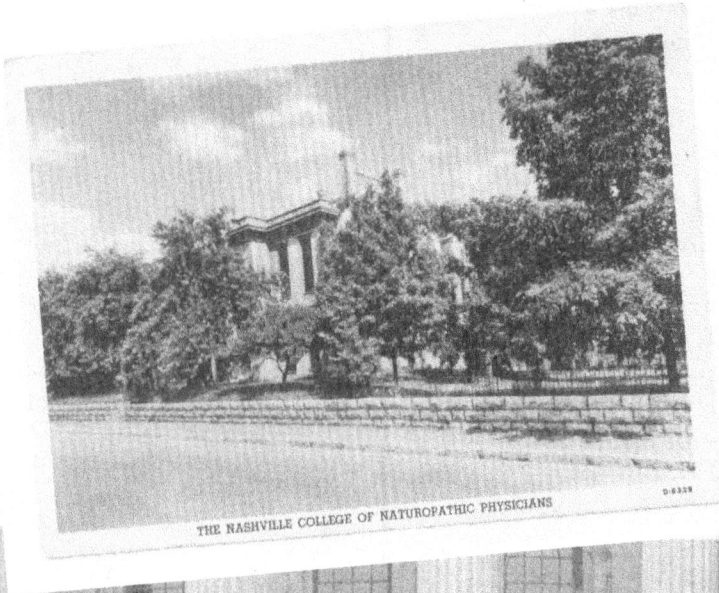

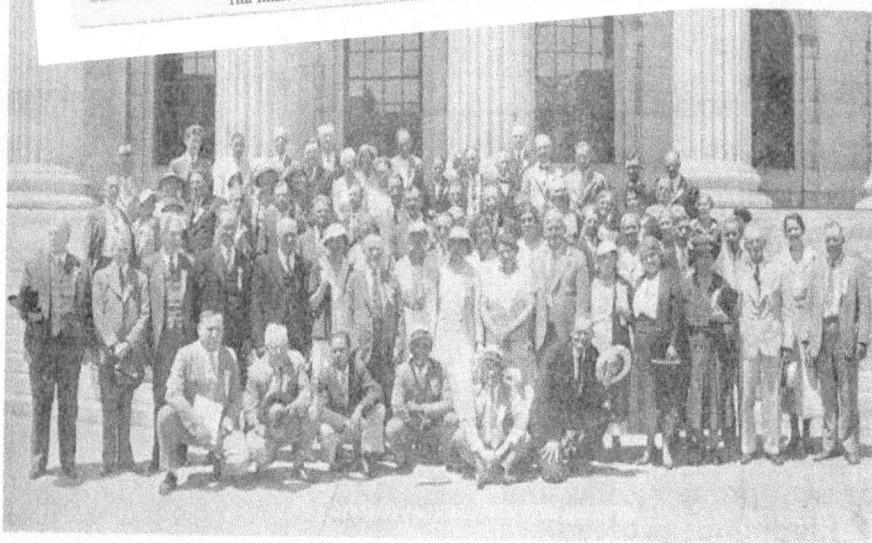

In California, where the right to practice was hard-fought and won in 1922, and the public embraced drugless methods readily, attempts to rescind the practice act failed. So the opponents of naturopaths and chiropractors simply solicited a legal opinion as to what the scope of practice entailed. By interpreting the methods very narrowly, it might be possible to put the irregulars out of business if they could not avail themselves of all the therapies they so famously used.

Complicating the situation was the fact that those in the "straight" chiropractic community (who were not also naturopaths) were only too happy to see the "mixer" chiropractors and naturopaths reined in. Harry Finkel, ND, DC reported the situation:

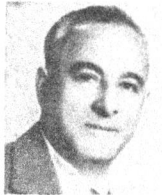

"...They intended to prove that the bill did not permit the use of all drugless methods, regardless of whether it was so stated in the bill in very simple language, and to have it declared illegal. Arrests of a few prominent natural healers were instituted with a view of making a test case. Two cases were tried in the lower court, and the instigators won both decisions.

"Judge James, of San Jose, before whom one of the cases was heard, defined Chiropractic as being the adjustment of the twenty-four vertebrae of the spinal column only, and that Chiropractors or Naturopaths have no legal right to use physiotherapy (electric treatments), hydrotherapy (water treatments), hygiene or diet, and in fact a drugless doctor is henceforth not permitted to tell his patients to eat whole wheat bread, take a sun bath, exercise, or even give or advise an enema." (Harry Finkel, ND, DC; *The Naturopath,* October 1934)

THE NASHVILLE COLLEGE OF NATUROPATHIC PHYSICIANS

The Officers and Delegates of the 38th Annual Congress of the American Naturopathic Association held at Hotel Albany, Denver, Colorado, May 31st, June 1st, 2nd and 3rd, 1934.

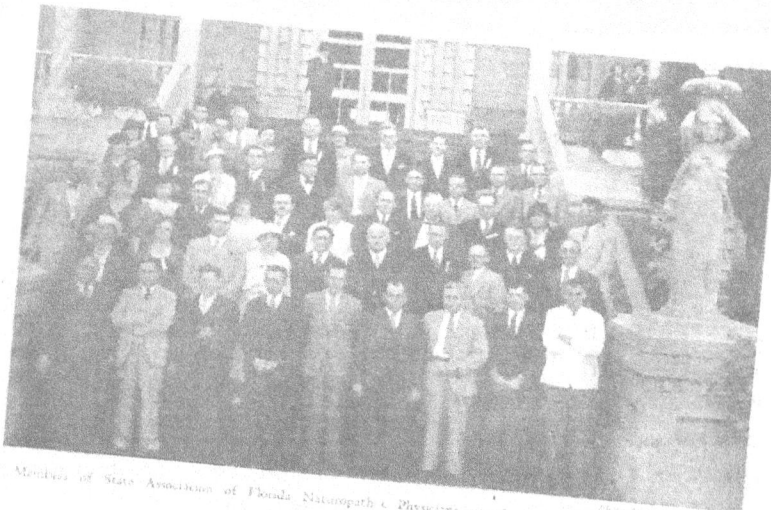

Members of State Association of Florida Naturopathic Physicians attend clinic at Centro Espanol Hospital

1935–

•**Dr. Robert V. Carroll**, president of the Washington State Naturopathic Association, presided at a meeting in Portland, Oregon, on "the unification and coordination of Naturopathy and Chiropractic". Two months later, Dr. Benedict Lust objects to this, saying "Let us say right here and now that we are against any alliance between naturopaths and chiropractors... Whenever we have ventured to co-operate with this crew we have gone down to defeat because they confuse the issues to our irreparable harm. Let them go their way and we'll go ours." *

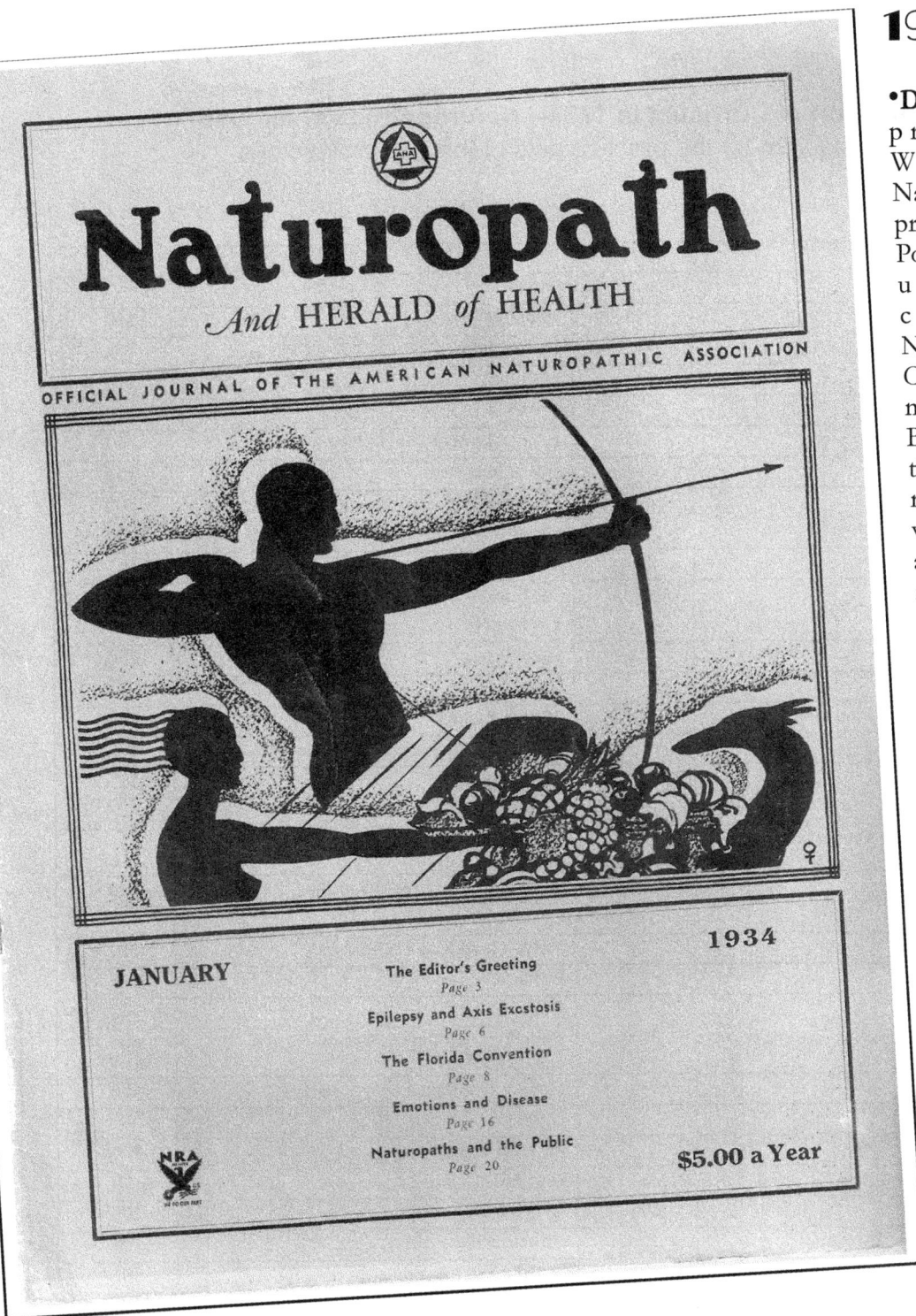

Naturopath

And HERALD *of* HEALTH

OFFICIAL JOURNAL OF THE AMERICAN NATUROPATHIC ASSOCIATION

1934

JANUARY

The Editor's Greeting
Page 3

Epilepsy and Axis Exostosis
Page 6

The Florida Convention
Page 8

Emotions and Disease
Page 16

Naturopaths and the Public
Page 20

$5.00 a Year

NRA

* February 1935 issue of *Naturopath*

Comparison of Curricula in 1934—Naturopathic vs. Allopathic
As required by the practice acts of the two professions

NATUROPATHIC	Hours	ALLOPATHIC	Hours
Group 1:		Group 1:	
Chemistry	145	Anatomy	550
Biology	145	Embryology	75
Physics	145	Histology	150
Group 2:		Group 2:	
Anatomy	485	Elem. Chemistry/toxicology	140
Histology	115	Adv. Chemistry	180
		Physiology	300
Group 3:		Group 3:	
Physiology	200	Elem. Bacteriology	60
		Adv. Bacteriology	80
		Hygiene	60
		Pathology	250
Group 4:		Group 4:	
Pathology, Bacteriology, Immunology	400	Materia medica	80
		Pharmacology	105
		Therapeutics	55
Group 5:		Group 5:	
Toxicology, Hygiene, Preventative medicine	120	Dermatology & Syphilis	45
		General Medicine & Diagnosis	600
		Genitourinary Diseases	45
		Nervous and Mental Diseases	110
		Pediatrics	140
Group 6:		Group 6:	
Biochemistry, Phytotherapy & Dietetics	240	Rhinology, Otology, Laryngology, Ophthalmology	60
		Surgery & Surgical Diagnosis	500
		Orthopedic Surgery	30
		Physical Therapy	30
Group 7:		Group 7:	
Minor Surgery	200	Gynecology	100
Anaesthesiology	50	Obstetrics	165
Group 8:		Jurisprudence & Ethics	30
Diagnosis	400		
Group 9:			
Naturopathic pathology, Theory & Practice, Physiotherapy, Hydrotherapy, Electrotherapy, Mechanotherapy, Suggestive therapy and Applied Psychology	500		
Clinic	190		
Group 10:			
Gynecology	100		
Obstetrics (incl. 15 bedside cases)	165		
TOTAL HOURS	3600	TOTAL HOURS	4000

1935—

- **Sophie B. Scheel, MD, dies.** She was a homeopathic physician and first Vice-president of the ANA. She was the first to suggest "Naturopathy" as a name for the field.

- **Arizona licenses** naturopathic doctors to practice.

- **Carl Schultz, ND, dies at 85.** Known as the "Father of Naturopathy on the West Coast", he was born in Germany. He was one of the original graduates of Lust's American School of Naturopathy in New York. Schultz was President Emeritus of the California University of Liberal Physicians and President of the Naturopathic Institute of California.

- Newly-chartered **University of the Healing Arts** in Hartford, Connecticut has three colleges, one of Naturopathy, one of Chiropractic, and one of physiotherapy. Dr. Per Nelson is Dean.

- **Columbia College of Naturopathy** inaugurates their four-year program on September 9th. Graduates will be offered internship at a Naturopathic sanitarium.

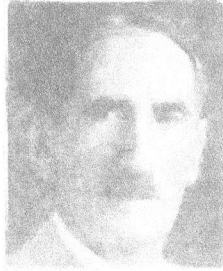

In 1935, the constitution and by-laws of the American Naturopathic Association were re-written by Dr. Robert Carroll at Dr. Benedict Lust's request. The ANA Board of Directors approved the new rules, which were signed into life at the annual ANA convention (this year in Omaha, Nebraska). Since accepting the office of "President-for-life" in 1922, Lust had delegated responsibility in the organization to a number of capable people, and these individuals now had a degree of power in both the national organization and also in the state associations. Robert Carroll, in particular, would become a major figure in the course of naturopathic history in the next decade because of his trusted status. Drafting the new by-laws in 1935 was only a harbinger of the new Naturopathy he would design. While serving in responsible positions in the national organization, Carroll and others would soon seek to depose the directors of the American Naturopathic Association and claim the organization as their own.

Meanwhile, Naturopathy is doing well in other parts of the world in 1935.

- **British College of Naturopathy** (later British College of Naturopathy and Osteopathy) is established by Stanley Leif, ND. Leif trained in the U.S. and was originally dispatched to England by Bernarr MacFadden to run a nature cure resort MacFadden had created. Later, Leif would set up a naturopathic clinic and resort that would become world-famous— *Champney's*, located in the former Rothschild mansion at Tring, Hertfordshire.

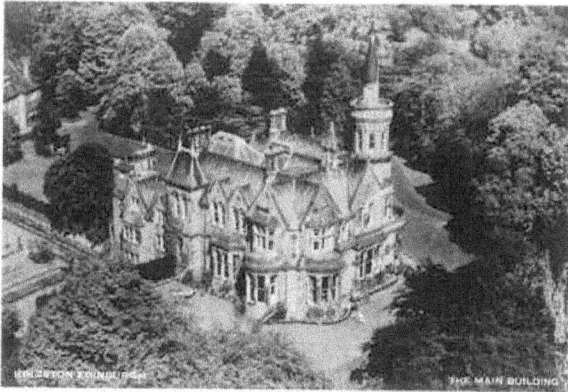

James C. Thomson, ND founded this other famous nature cure establishment in the United Kingdom, **Kingston Clinic** in Edinburgh. Thomson studied under Henry Lindlahr in America, and founded the Edinburgh School of Natural Therapeutics.

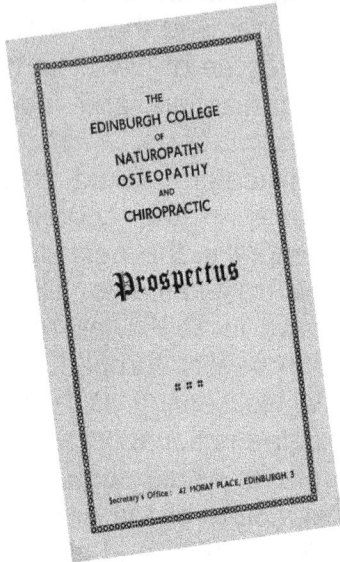

THE
EDINBURGH COLLEGE
OF
NATUROPATHY
OSTEOPATHY
AND
CHIROPRACTIC

Prospectus

* * *

Secretary's Office: 42 MORAY PLACE, EDINBURGH 3

1936—

- **Naturopathic Practice Act becomes law** in British Columbia, Canada.

- The November issue of *Scientific Chiropractor*, (Vol. 1, No. 4) contains this news item:

TEST FIGHT ON THERAPY LAW IN CALIFORNIA FAILS
Highest Court Will Leave Question of Naturopathic Practice Up To State

Washington, Oct. 14 (AP)—Whether the practice of Naturopathy by a group of Chiropractors in California should be permitted was left today by the Supreme Court to State officials to determine.

The court refused to review a ruling April 12, 1935, by the Southern Federal District Court of California that the dispute presented no federal question.

The California Medical Practice and Chiropractic Acts were called unconstitutional by the United States Naturopathic Association, Ltd., its officers, and individual members.

It listed headquarters at Phoenix, Ariz., and a branch at Hollywood and asked an injunction against the Chiropractic League of California, State Board of Examiners, and State officials to prevent them from "arresting and interfering with" the naturopaths, who are also chiropractors.

BAR SUIT ON CHIROPRACTIC LEAGUE

The Supreme Court refused to consider the $1,000,000 suit of the United States Naturopathic Association, Ltd., against the Chiropractic League of California. California Attorney General US Webb, and the State Board of Chiropractic Examiners.

The naturopathic healers contended in a suit against the Chiropractic group that the latter had conspired to bar them from the practice of their profession in California.

- **Paul Bragg, ND**, noted health lecturer, was arrested in Washington D.C. Newspapers read "Teacher is arrested who has done $50,000,000 worth of damage to the medical profession." Bragg had been drawing large audiences all over the country, and was charged with violating the Medical Practice Act of the District of Columbia. He was released on bail and when his case came to trial, he was fined $100.

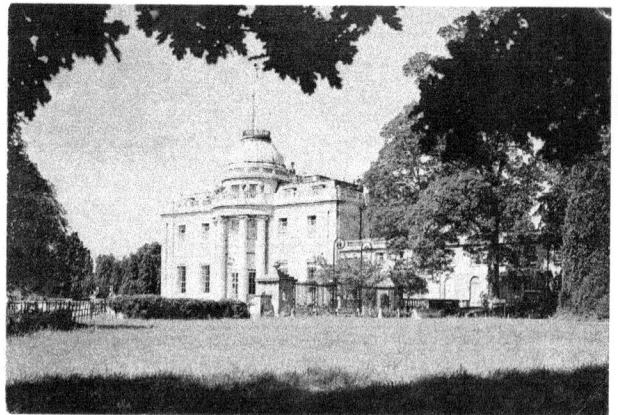

Tyringham Naturopathic Clinic, England

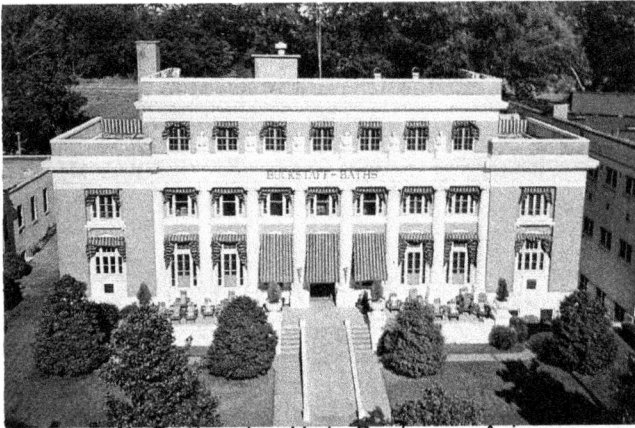

Buckstaff Baths in Hot Springs, Arizona—a hydrotherapy Mecca on this side of the Atlantic.

1936—

- **A two-day meeting of the executive committee of the American Naturopathic Association** was held in June, at which Dr. Benedict Lust expressed his desire to resign as President. He had expressed a similar request in 1921, but there was unanimous opposition to it at that time, and the members then elected him as Life President. Now, he said, he was weary of financing the ANA, as member dues were not supporting the organization, and that he had received uncomplimentary letters over the last year that the Executive Committee agreed did not show him the respect due as president. Acting chairman of the meeting, Dr. Robert V. Carroll, asked that the committee not consider the resignation, and that he "trusts and hopes that all the past of any grievance and ill feeling and lack of consideration of any of the members be forgiven." Dr. F.R. Good explained his reasons for writing some of the offending correspondence and apologized. The Executive Committee was composed of: Dr. Lust, President; Dr. T.M. Schippell, Corresponding Secretary; Dr. T. Louise Nedvidek, Financial Secretary; Dr. George Colingwood, Covention Manager; Dr. Robert V. Carroll, Dr. L.A. Lyons; Dr. F.R. Good; Dr. A.C. Pusheck.

- **New York State steps up its persecution of naturopaths** during the summer, arresting four NDs in three months for practicing medicine without a license. Two of them would be prominent figures of the movement: Herbert Shelton and Max Warmbrand. William Meyer was also arrested, and Jacob Levine, whose "crime" was giving a series of lectures on Iridology. Benedict Lust, in *Naturopath and Herald of Health*, said, "We warn the powers that be that this persecution must cease." He pointed out that "A naturopath or chiropractor who is convicted a third time of practicing in New York can be sentenced to nineteen years in the penitentiary and ordered to pay a big fine. This equals the sentence that may be imposed for second degree murder."*

- **Naturopath Dr. Carl Frischkorn demonstrates amazing success in treating infantile paralysis (polio)** with natural means. In addition to his own practice, he canvasses the United States and finds that not one case resulted in paralysis when treated naturopathically first. Dr. Frischkorn's methods do not differ substantially from the later "Sister Kenny Treatment", which would become world-famous.

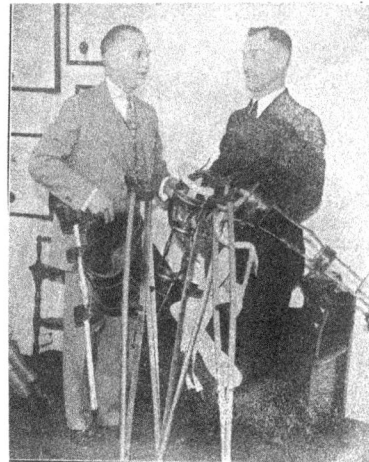

Dr. Frischkorn (left) and his associate Dr. Phillips with the growing pile of braces, crutches, and other appliances discarded by cured polio patients.

1937—

- **S o u t h C a r o l i n a l i c e n s e s** naturopathic doctors.

- **Naturopathic hospital** is established in B e z w a d a , India.

The Drugless Hospital, Bezwada.
Conducted under the personal superintendence of
Dr. K. W. BHAIRAVAMURTY, B.A., N.D.,
(President, Indian Naturopathic Association.)

Bezwada town lies on the northern bank of the River Krishna. The Hospital is located in a building outside the town, in sanitary and peaceful surroundings near the river bank. There is also an open air Sanitarium attached to the Hospital, lying within two furlongs from the Hospital and situated in a mango grove in the very river bed. With the river flowing closely and mountains all round, the natural scenery surrounding the sanitarium is charming and exhilarating. In-patients of the Hospital, after a certain improvement, may, if they so desire, be transferred to the sanitarium on suitable terms.

The Hospital provides efficient Naturopathic Treatment for all diseases, Chronic and Acute. The harmlessness of Naturopathic remedies, and the certainty and permanence of the cures effected by them, are well-known,

---

* *Naturopath and Herald of Health,* May 1936, p. 132; August 1936, p. 249.

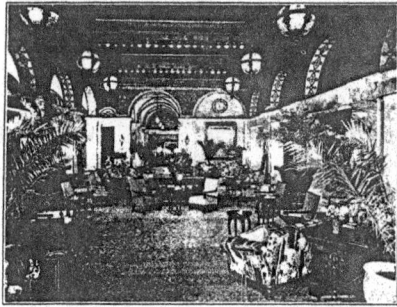

Lobby of Congress Hotel, Chicago, Ill.

The 41st Annual Convention

of the

AMERICAN NATUROPATHIC ASSOCIATION
September 22nd, 23rd, 24th, 25th, 26th, 1937

at the

Congress Hotel — Chicago, Illinois

The American Naturopathic Association is going right ahead with its plans for the greatest Convention ever held under its auspices. No city in the country is so well equipped as Chicago for this purpose. It is centrally located and quickly accessible from all parts of the country. Practitioners from all over the country and many foreign ones have indicated their intention of being present at the Association's Forty-First Congress.

The lectures, demonstrations, clinics, special and post-graduate courses this year will be on an extremely high level. Many of the most prominent men and women in the profession are on the tentative program.

Make your plans NOW to attend. Don't let anything stop you!

For further information, watch future issues of the "Naturopath" and "Nature's Path" — or write to

Dr. T. Louise Nedvidek
CONVENTION MANAGER

620 CAMERON AVENUE   LA CROSSE, WISCONSIN

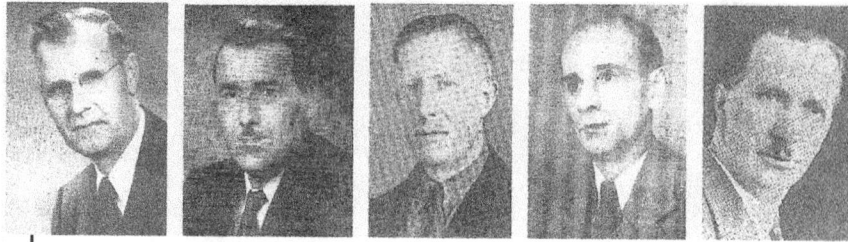

ISNP officers Schramm (USA), Campanella (USA), Bodewin (Canada), Schonderlein (Germany), and Orbell (England)

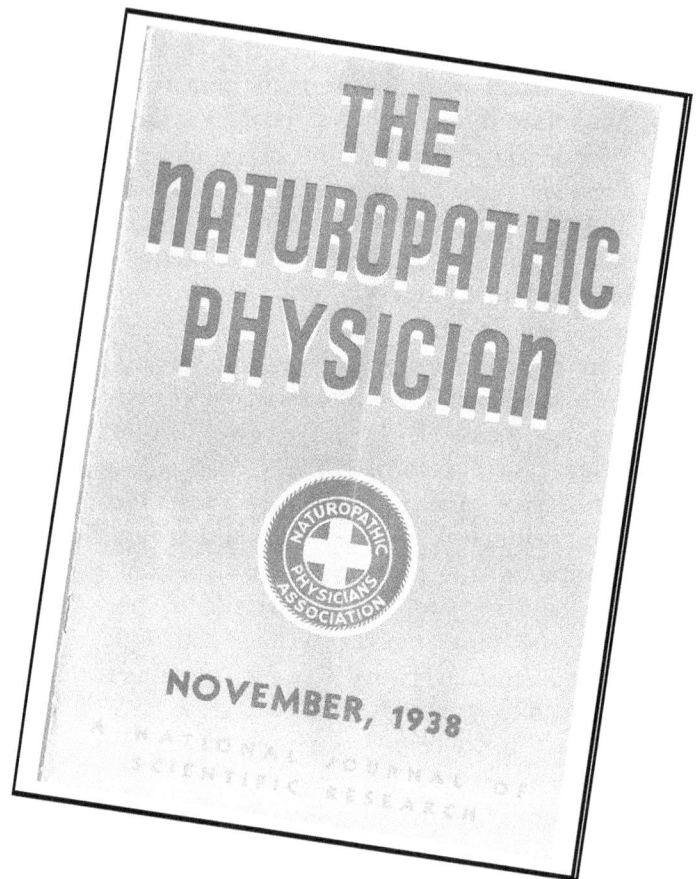

THE NATUROPATHIC PHYSICIAN

NOVEMBER, 1938

A NATIONAL JOURNAL OF SCIENTIFIC RESEARCH

1938—

- **John Scheel, MD, dies** in June of 1938. He and his wife Sophie Scheel, MD, sold the rights to the term "Naturopathy" to Benedict Lust in 1902, beginning a cohesive form for the developing synthesis of Nature Cure methods under Lust's hand.

- **The International Society of Naturopathic Physicians is formed.** The first organization with an international scope, it becomes popular with both basic "nature cure" advocates and progressive naturopathic physicians, and coordinates communication among practitioners in many countries. Founders include Drs. Arthur Schramm, Peter Spelio, Harold Foster, Hugh Aitchinson, W.J. Maxwell, Edward Shook, Evelyn Burkholder, and Malcolm Mackintosh[*].

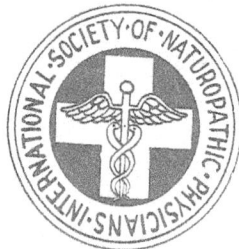

---

[*] Schramm, A.C., *ISNP Archives,* Los Angeles

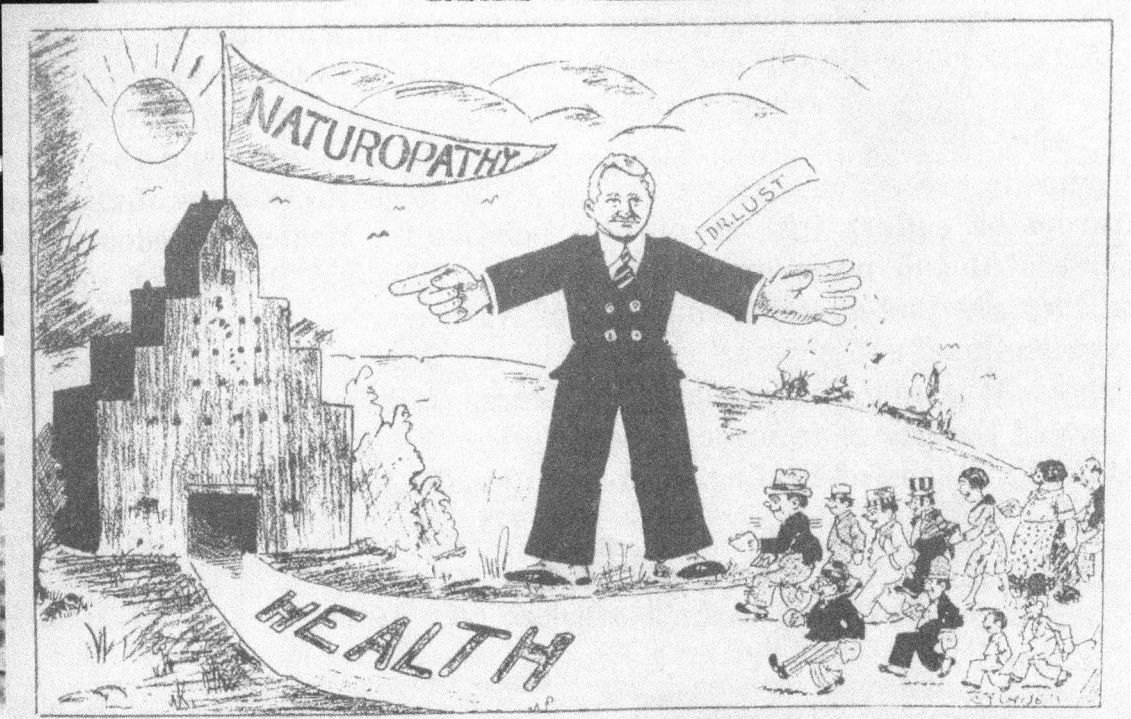

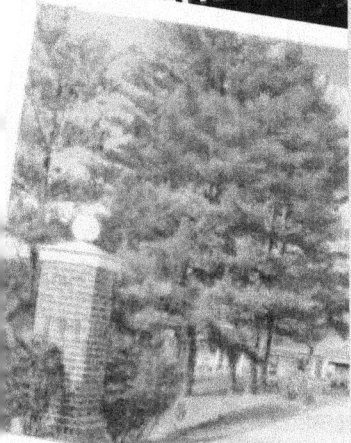

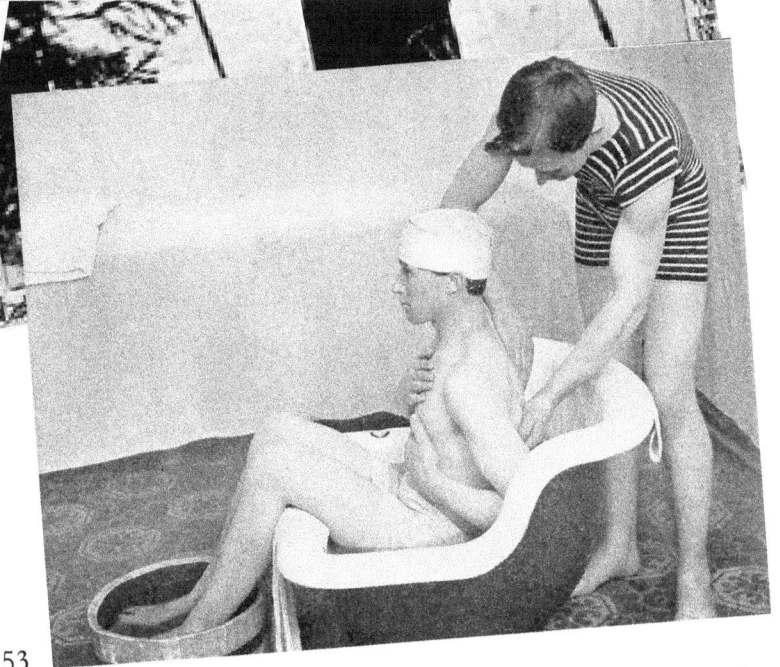

1939—

- **Dr. Herbert Shelton** begins publishing *The Hygienic Review*, a monthly magazine that would run over 40 years.

- **Utah licenses** naturopathic doctors.

- **The New York World's Fair bars exhibits** of naturopathic, osteopathic, chiropractic, naprapathic, dietetic, and physiotherapy methods. Only orthodox medicine is represented in the "World of Tomorrow" exhibit. Dr. Benedict Lust decries this monopolistic gesture, saying "We would rather have it called 'The World of Yesterday'."

- **Southern California College of Chiropractic opens its College of Naturopathy**, offering a postgraduate course to chiropractors and a 4000-hour course of instruction including "colonic, electro-, and fever therapy, hospital internship and clinics."

- On April 24th, police and representatives of the California State Medical Board entered the Alta Vista Hospital, a naturopathic institution, and served **arrest warrants for Edward Shook, ND and Evelyn Burkholder, ND.** The officers searched the premises without a search warrant, claiming they were "looking for morphine". Dr. Shook was not allowed to phone his attorney. Equipment and records were taken, and the two doctors taken to jail. A jury trial of practicing medicine without a license was held in July, ending in a mistrial. A second trial was held and the two naturopaths were acquitted.

A POPULAR GUIDE TO NATURE CURE
By V. Stanley Davidson, N.D., D.O., D.C., D.A.

NATUROPATHY OSTEOPATHY
CHIROPRACTIC HYDROTHERAPY
HOMEOPATHY

The eclectic character of Nature Cure is evident in this illustration. All the drugless healing methods were finding a focal point with Naturopathy.

The
JOURNAL *of* DRUGLESS PHYSICIANS

TO ADVANCE THE
COMITY BETWEEN AND
AMONG ALL DIVISIONS
OF THE HEALING ARTS

Vol. 2   MARCH 1940   No. 2

1939— (continued)

Central States College of Physiatrics is chartered and opens in Eaton, Ohio, near Columbus. It is founded by Harry Riley Spitler, PhD, MD, ND. It quickly becomes approved as an educational institution by the American Naturopathic Association.

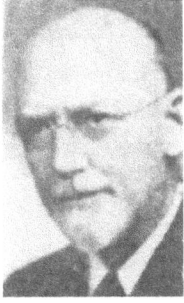

"Physiatrics" was not a commonly-used term in 1939. Spitler applied it to his program because naturopaths were not specifically licensed in Ohio, and opposition to such was so strong that it was never likely to happen. However, mechanotherapists were licensable. Central's Mechanotherapy program was nearly identical in content to the curricula of colleges of Naturopathy. In effect, naturopaths were licensed in Ohio as mechanotherapists, and Spitler used this to good advantage, since he learned that the medical lobby was unable to eliminate the Mechanotherapy profession and did not want an influx of even more irregular practitioners into the state if they licensed naturopaths. As a result, Central States' program was a bit more comprehensive than other Mechanotherapy courses, covering the breadth of naturopathic practice and making its graduates very competitive in the field. Graduates who were bound for other states could be awarded the ND degree rather than the in-state Doctor of Mechanotherapy. The school was also known as **Central States College of Naturopathy**.

Central States' courses in botanical medicine were used by other venues; for example, the State of Florida required that its ND licensees must have had training in it. Graduates of schools that did not require botanical medicine courses had to travel to Ohio to get their certificate in order to qualify for their Florida licenses.

Spitler himself was a mutli-faceted individual. Having trained in light and color therapy under Dr. Carl Loeb, one of the top experts in the field, Spitler combined this knowledge with Optometry and founded the postgraduate College of Syntonic Optometry (still in existence today as a source of instruction in vision-training and brain re-mapping therapy).

In 1948, Spitler would go on to write a major textbook, *Basic Naturopathy*.

- Following the publication of the book *Return To Eden* by Jethro Kloss, the Tennessee State Medical Association put pressure on the publisher to advertise only that the book was for sale, but not to advertise any of its contents. Since the book advised the reader how to use natural therapeutics and was a compendium of the medical uses of common herbs, the book was not to be used "for any therapeutic purpose". Later, the Tennessee legislature would make the practice of natural medicine a "gross misdemeanor", punishable by up to one year in jail.

- **Germany passes a law recognizing and regulating naturopathic practitioners.** The *Heilpraktikergesetz* ("health practitioners law") requires basic science training.

Meanwhile, **Bernarr MacFadden** (Called "Public Enemy Number One" by Morris Fishbein, President of the American Medical Association) continues to establish his "Physical Culture hotels" throughout America. These institutions were a combination of naturopathic sanitarium and vacation health resort. One of the most famous was in Dansville, New York. It had previously been known as "Our Home on the Hill" when owned and operated by James Caleb Jackson, MD.

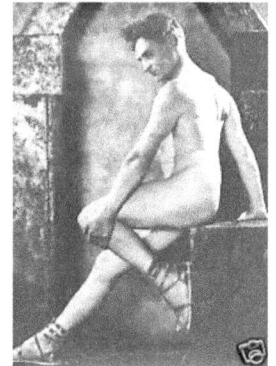

Jackson ran a private sanitarium there for many years, using only drugless methods. Jackson also authored some early nature cure books. While much has been written about James Harvey Kellogg of the Battle Creek Sanitarium originating corn flakes, Jackson actually created the first dry breakfast cereal in 1863. He called it "Granula".

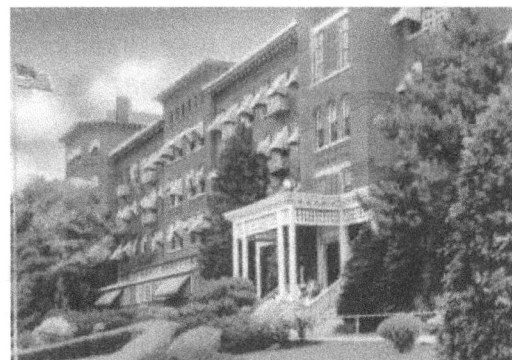

Bernarr MacFadden, a naturopath called "Public Enemy Number One" by the President of the American Medical Association

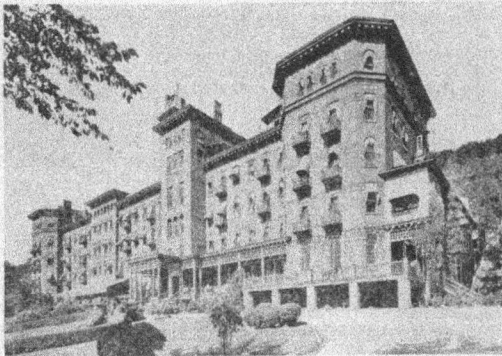

Bernarr MacFadden's fame was due not only to his string of health resorts, but to his flamboyant personality infusing the many magazines and books he published: *Physical Culture* and other health-related titles, plus *Photoplay, True Story, True Detective, Amazing Stories,* and many other popular magazines of the day. He would write over 100 books in his lifetime. Since MacFadden owned a publishing empire, he was hard to silence. While health lecturers like Paul Bragg were routinely arrested, MacFadden was able to keep the natural medicine message before the American public in a way that no one else could. Benedict Lust considered him a valuable ally, and MacFadden's "Physcultopathy" (as he named it) was seen as a worthy subset of Naturopathy by Lust.

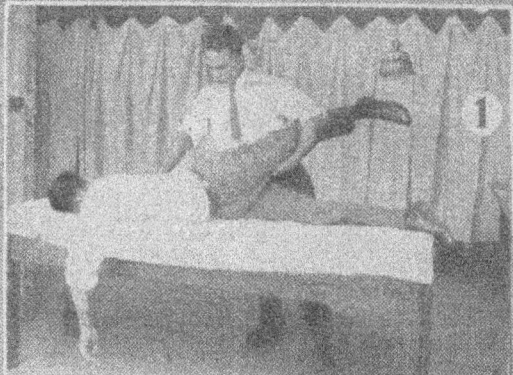
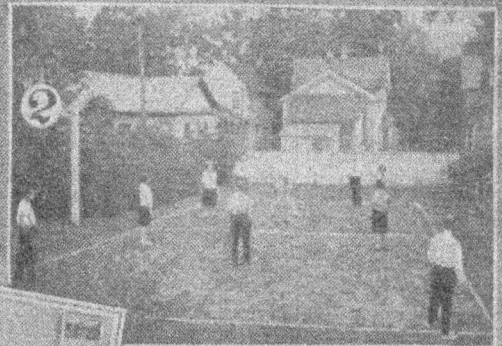
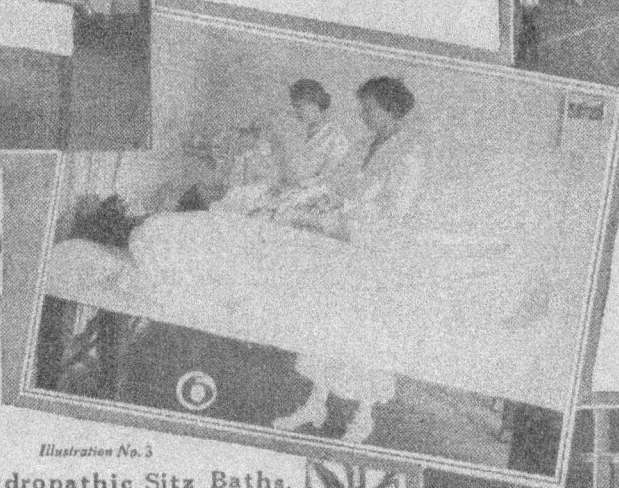
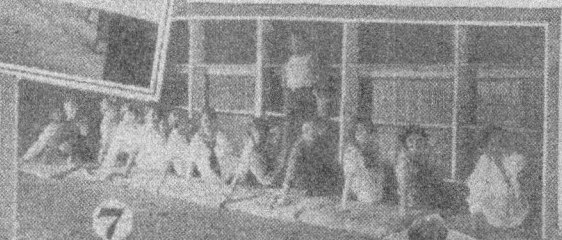
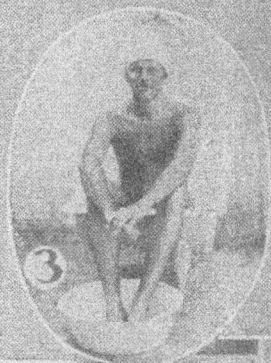
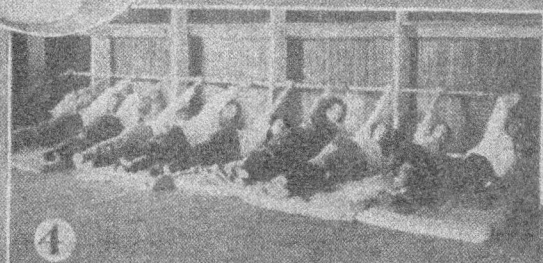
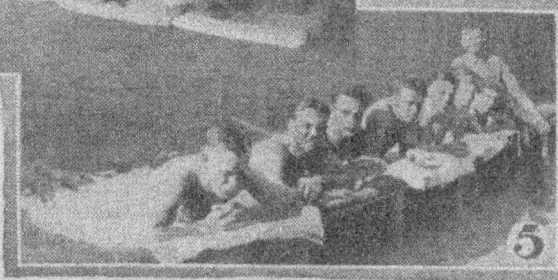
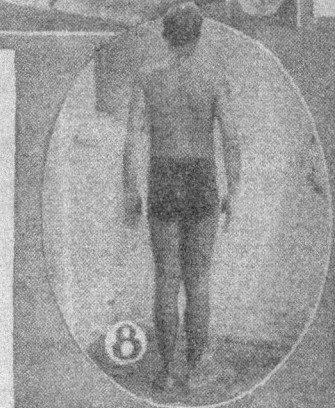
57

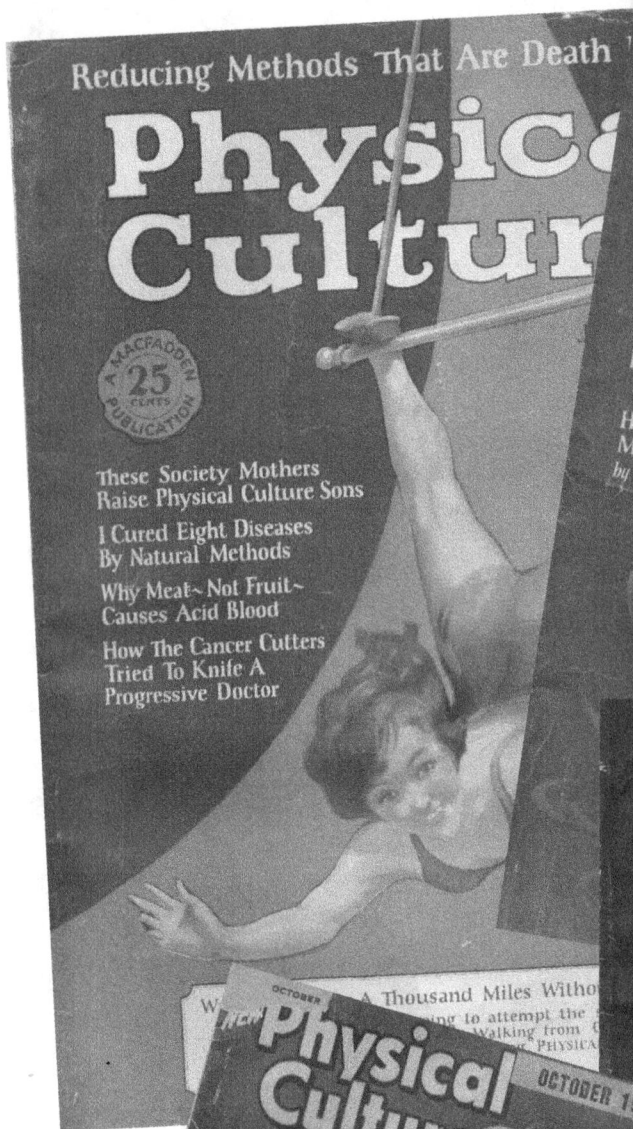

Reducing Methods That Are Death...

Physical Culture

A MACFADDEN PUBLICATION
25 CENTS

These Society Mothers
Raise Physical Culture Sons

I Cured Eight Diseases
By Natural Methods

Why Meat~Not Fruit~
Causes Acid Blood

How The Cancer Cutters
Tried To Knife A
Progressive Doctor

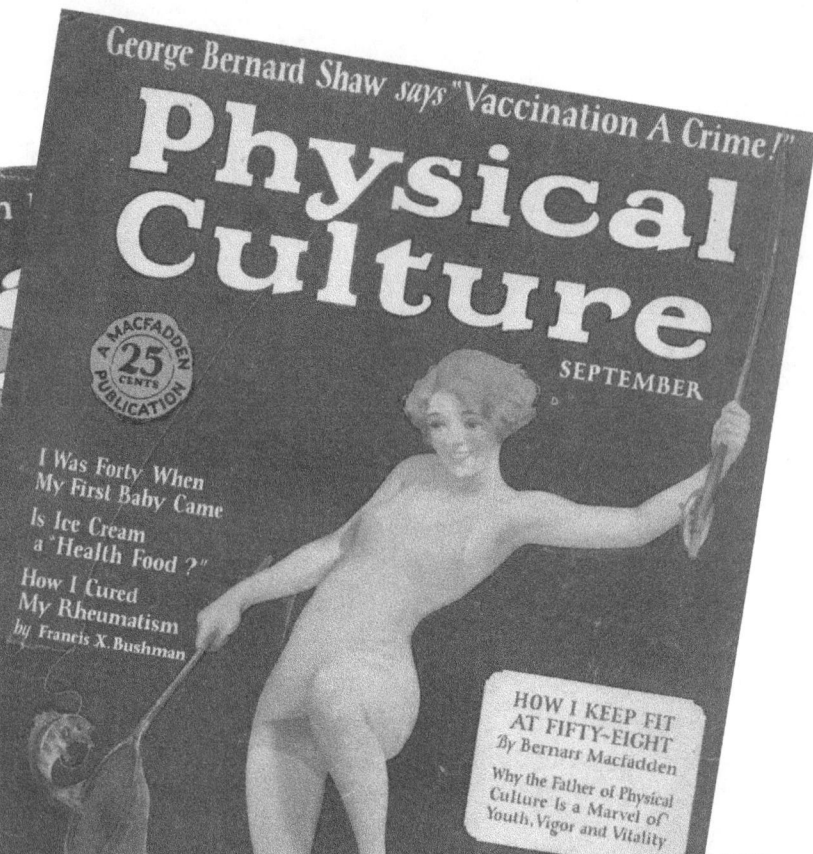

George Bernard Shaw *says* "Vaccination A Crime!"

Physical Culture

SEPTEMBER

A MACFADDEN PUBLICATION
25 CENTS

I Was Forty When
My First Baby Came

Is Ice Cream
a "Health Food?"

How I Cured
My Rheumatism
by Francis X. Bushman

HOW I KEEP FIT
AT FIFTY~EIGHT
By Bernarr Macfadden

Why the Father of Physical
Culture Is a Marvel of
Youth, Vigor and Vitality

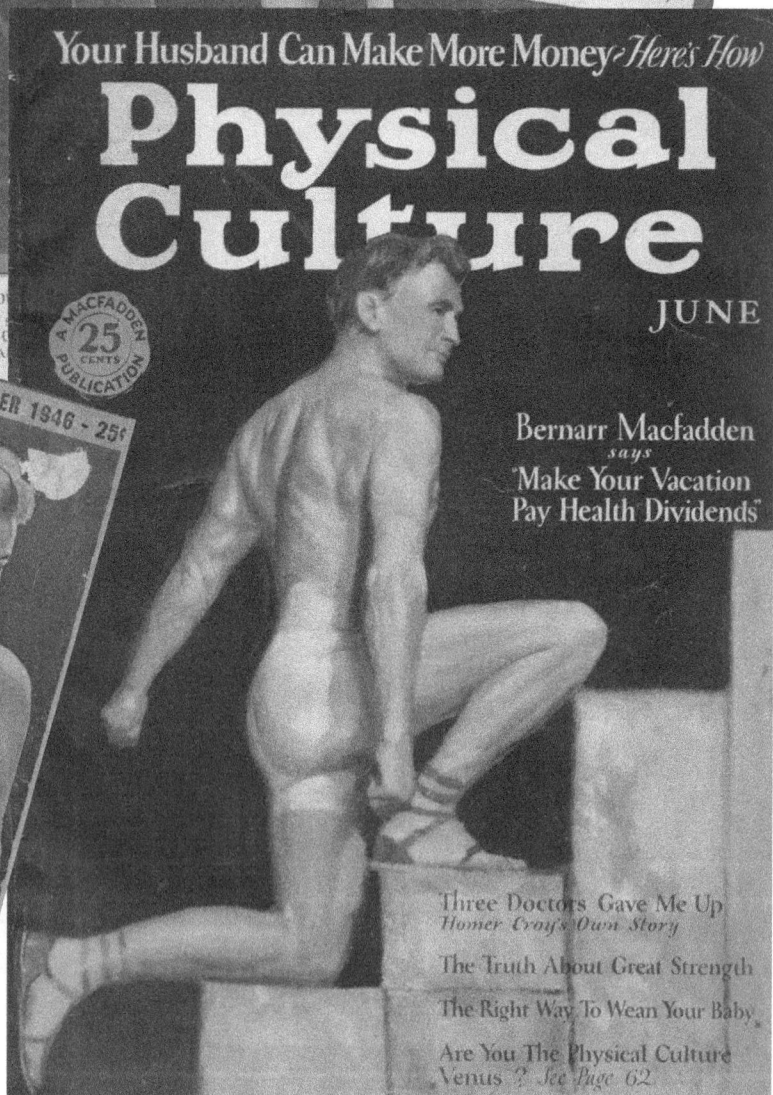

OCTOBER ... A Thousand Miles Witho...
...ing to attempt the ...
Walking from ...

NEW Physical Cultur...

OCTOBER 1946 - 25¢

MARVELOUS...
GRAPE DIET
FOR CANCER

Your Husband Can Make More Money~*Here's How*

Physical Culture

JUNE

A MACFADDEN PUBLICATION
25 CENTS

Bernarr Macfadden
says
"Make Your Vacation
Pay Health Dividends"

Three Doctors Gave Me Up
Homer Croy's Own Story

The Truth About Great Strength

The Right Way To Wean Your Baby

Are You The Physical Culture
Venus? *See Page* 62

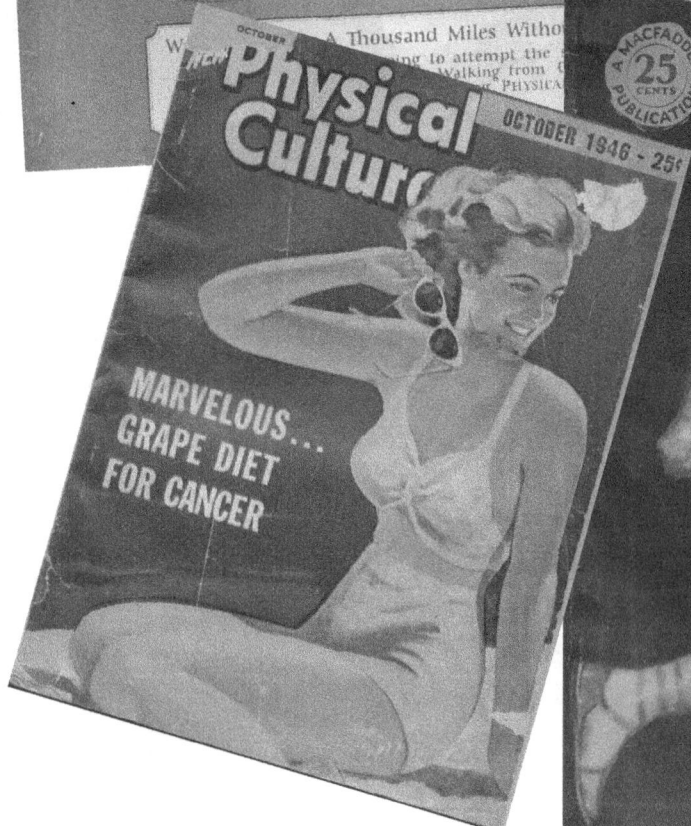

1940—

- **National Board of Naturopathic Examiners is established.** Each state continues to have its own board of examiners, however.

- **Florida naturopaths win an important legal decision** in November 1940. Although licensed in that state since 1927, in 1939 the State Board of Health forced them to rescind a rule that allowed them to obtain human specimens and order laboratory tests. From that time, only medical doctors, osteopaths, and dentists were legally able to do so. The Florida Supreme Court ruled that a school of medicine licensed by the state could not be discriminated against, and overruled motions by the Attorney General and the Board of Health to quash the new Writ of Alternative Mandamus. NDs now assumed a greater degree of parity with other doctors.

- Ground is broken in the summer for the new **College of Naturopathy** in Centerville, Michigan. Founded and partially funded by McKinney Brothers Sanitarium, it expects an enrollment of 200, and will boast a faculty of 15 full time professors and a host of associate professors.

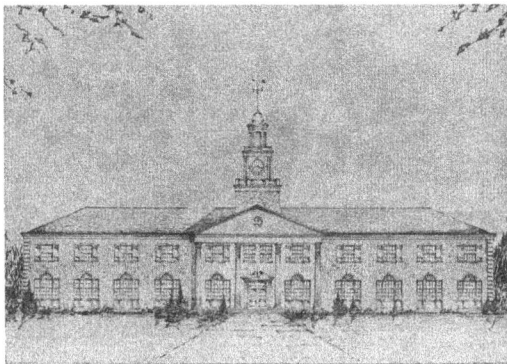

Proposed Centerville College

A dormitory for 50 students will be located on the upper floor. The Naturopathic Association of Michigan has 280 members, and has around 200 applications for training from several states, insuring that the enrollment the first year should be nearly full capacity.

Naturopathy is moving briskly forward.

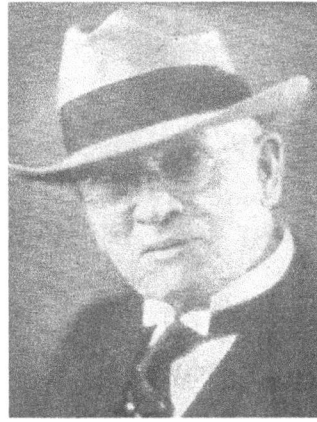

- **Dr. J.H. Tilden of Denver, Colorado dies at the age of 89.** One of the pioneers, he operated a nature cure sanitarium for decades and was the only doctor in Colorado who never had even one death from pneumonia. He was the author of *Toxemia Explained*.

- **T. Louise Nedvidek, ND** is a prominent female naturopath and an active organizer with the American Naturopathic Association. She would serve as program director for many of the ANA conferences, and ran a respected naturopathic sanitarium in Wisconsin for many years. A trusted confrere of Benedict Lust, she illustrated the equality that has always existed in the naturopathic profession. In an era when few women were allowed to ascend to any heights in any profession (least of all medicine), Dr. Nedvidek was one of many of her gender to display to the world the impartiality and benevolence that characterized Naturopathy as envisioned by Lust, Collins, and the other

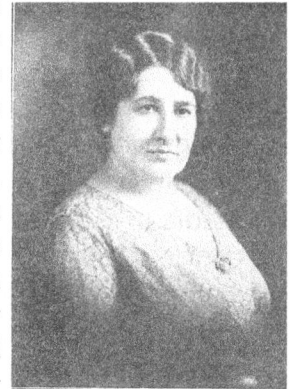

pioneers.

- **Robert V. Carroll, ND addressed the 44th Annual Congress of the ANA** in Chicago. He called for naturopaths to become standardized in their approach to diagnostic methods. Noting the "many divergences in naturopathic practice", he said "It is our duty as naturopaths to establish some kind of standardization in diagnosis and treatment in our profession."

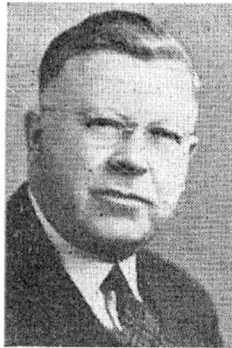

In a statement that is telling of the future direction Carroll and his followers would go, he said:

> "Many of our own doctors will accuse us of attempting to ape and imitate our medical kin by so conducting our office procedures. While we do take exception to the MD's principles, we must admire the confidence his "showmanship" and "front" have built up in the lay public. The best way to instill confidence in our patients is to show them that we have a *system of diagnosis* that is complete and second to none...we have not enough naturopaths who are systematized and standardized to such an extent that we could take over the Health Department of a single state and run it efficiently".

The implications of this speech will become clear in the next chapter; particularly the events to come in 1942, and the comments of Carroll's own brother, who would warn the profession of the coming movement to blend Naturopathy with orthodox medicine.

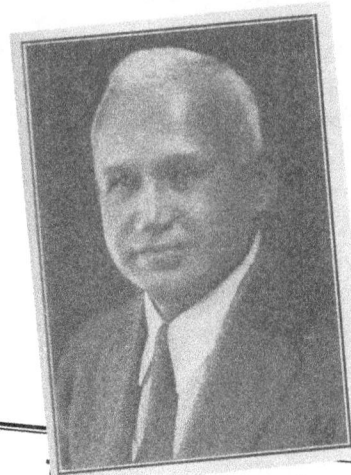

Dr. Lust's health resort, which would have a sister facility in Florida, was the model for many a Nature Cure establishment.

4

POLARIZATION

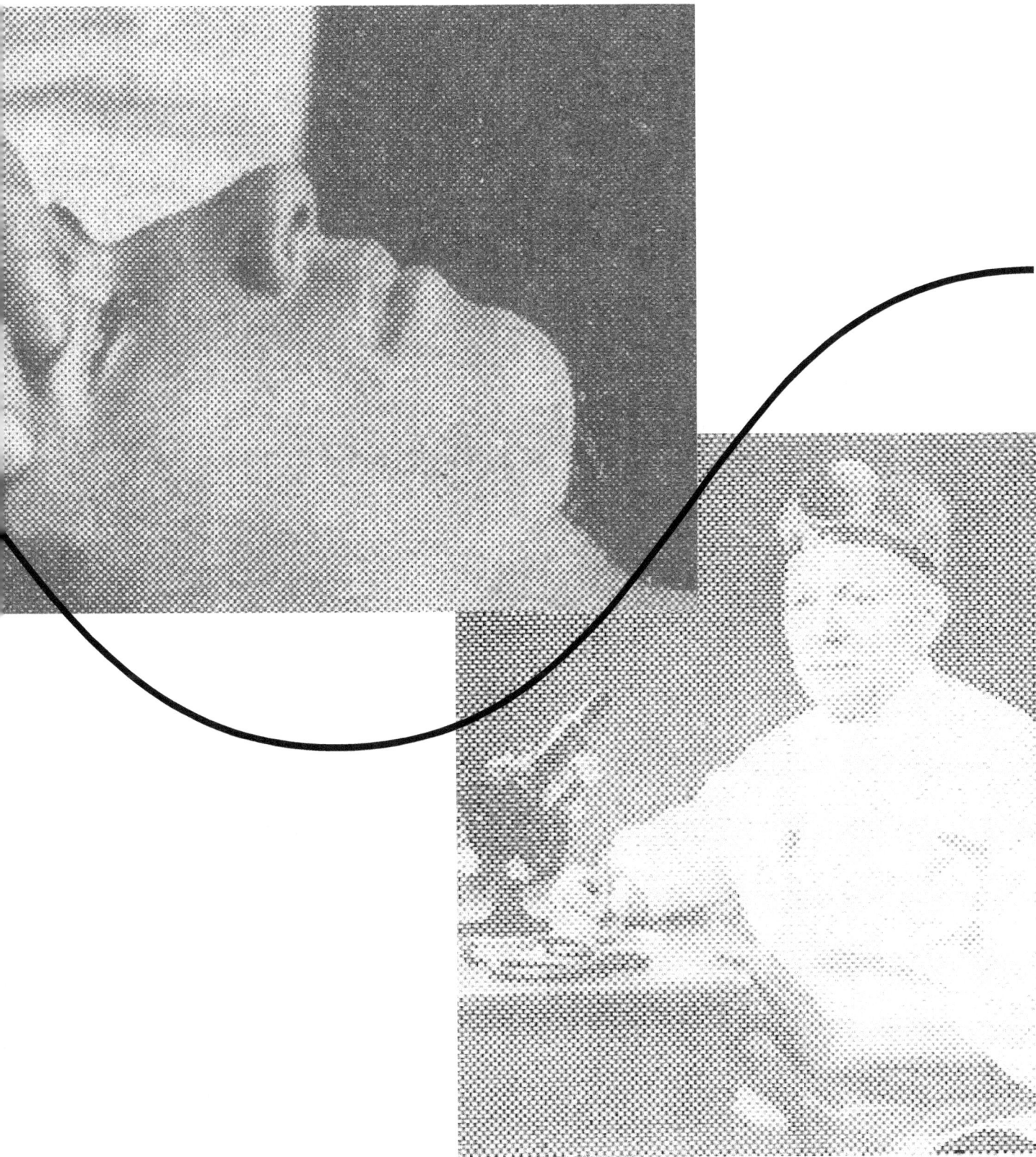

61

1941—

- **The American School of Naturopathy, Chicago branch, opens.** Dr. Benedict Lust serves as adjunct president.

- **Naturopathic doctors in Florida win** an important legal decision—the right to order diagnostic laboratory tests. A rule from 1939 granting access to only MDs, Dos, and dental surgeons was rescinded.

- **The naturopathic community begins polarizing, with some incorporating a greater number of diagnostic and treatment methods, and others taking a more fundamentalist stance.** Progressive naturopaths want to imitate conventional medicine in education and research, and conservatives insist on a purely "nature cure" approach.

- **Dr. Robert G. Jackson dies** at 84. A medical doctor who converted to Naturopathy, he wrote *How To Be Always Well*, and eight other books. He was the inventor of Roman Meal bread.

1942—

- **Lust's American School of Naturopathy in New York City closes.**

- **The U.S. Army buys the former Battle Creek Sanitarium**, making it the Percy Jones Army Hospital.

- *Physical Culture* **Magazine ceases publication.** The main voice of the Physical Culture movement, headed by Bernarr MacFadden, once had more than 400,000 subscribers. Dr. Jesse Mercer Gehman, Chairman of the ANA, points to the contrast between the petering out of this group and the continued growth of the naturopathic movement.

- A faction of naturopaths in the Northwest and Southwest states, which would come to be known as **the "Western Group", creates a second American Naturopathic Association.** This organization holds its own national convention in Chicago, undercutting attendance at the original ANA's convention in Atlantic City in June. The Western ANA is organized by Robert V. Carroll, Henry Schlichting, Jr., and Frederick Dugdale, who would be forever after referred to in naturopathic circles as "the renegades".*

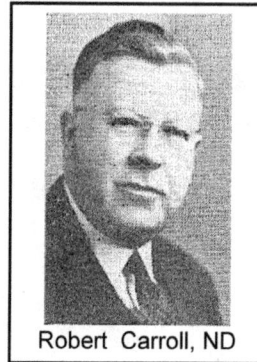

Robert Carroll, ND

Carroll becomes the first president of the new organization. Schlichting, of Midland, Texas, was a leader of what some called the "Midwestern Group", another band of dissidents who left the original ANA. Lust would later refer to him as "that self-appointed dictator".

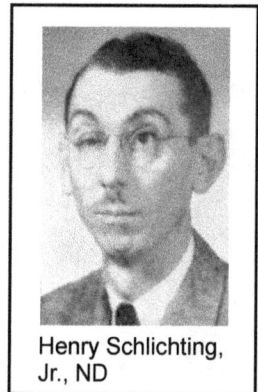

Henry Schlichting, Jr., ND

Schlichting and Carroll were both trusted by Benedict Lust and placed in positions of power. Their in-group raised the ANA membership dues dramatically, then used the increased revenue to build the Western organization, which they represented to members as the original and authentic American Naturopathic Association.

This audacious act sent the pioneering naturopaths reeling, not the least of whom was Dr. Lust himself. But the new faction attracted those who believed the promise of a progressive and more prestigious profession. Since the largest concentration of NDs were now in the Pacific Northwest (and still are, in the 21st Century), a large number of naturopaths gravitated to the Western ANA, which was governed by those in their own region, with Dr. Carroll at the helm.

* Kirchfeld, Friedhelm, and Wade Boyle. "Nature Doctors: Pioneers in Naturopathic Medicine". Medicina Biologica, 1994

1943–

- **Dr. John Harvey Kellogg dies** at 91. He ran the Battle Creek Sanitarium in Michigan for 50 years, the largest health institution in the world. In his later years, he ran another health resort in Florida, but it never achieved the success of his Battle Creek facility.

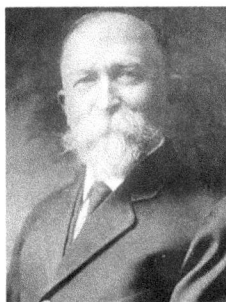

- **Jesse Mercer Gehman, ND** (several term ANA President) authors the book *Smoke Over America*, an early and prophetic examination of the dangers of tobacco smoke.

- **Fire destroys Benedict Lust's "Yungborn"** health resort in Florida. Dr. Lust is injured assisting the evacuation. No lives are lost. Arson is suspected.

- **Tennessee licenses** naturopathic doctors.

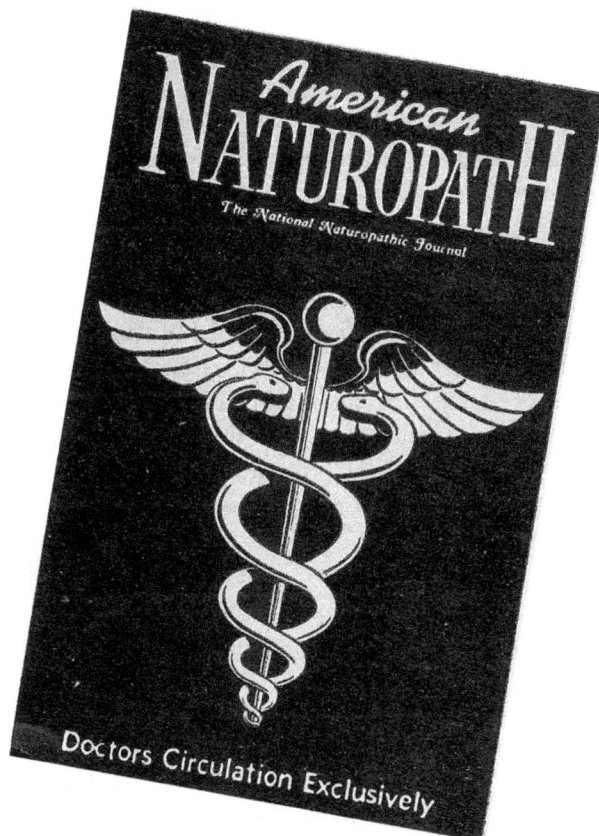

1944–

- Southern California College of Chiropractic establishes a sister institution, the **College of Naturopathic Physicians and Surgeons.** SCCC soon after will merge with Los Angeles Chiropractic College.

- **Thomas T. Lake, ND, writes** *Treatment of the Prostate by Physical and Manipulative Therapy.*

- **Virginia licenses** naturopathic doctors.

- **Publication begins** for *American Naturopath*, a digest-sized journal for the profession that would span decades. Carl Hotchkiss, ND, is editor.

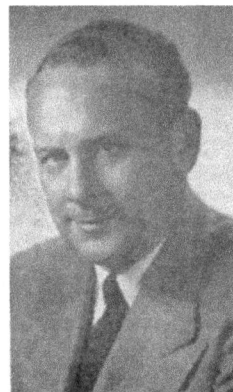

Carl Hotchkiss, ND

1945—

- **The Western "American Naturopathic Association" becomes a legal corporation.** It is populated by the progressives, referred to as "pseudo-medicalists" by the traditional naturopaths. Its president is H.A. Brown. The Eastern ANA likewise becomes incorporated, **resulting in two organizations known as "The American Naturopathic Association, Inc."** President Emeritus of the original ANA remains Benedict Lust.

- Lindlahr College of Natural Therapeutics is absorbed by National College of Chiropractic and renamed **National College of Drugless**

National College of Drugless Physicians

FOUR YEAR COURSE

Complete Structural Adjustment   Faculty of 21 Members
All Drugless Therapies   Internship with Pay
Superb Training Equipment

20 N. Ashland Blvd.   Chicago, Ill.

Physicians.

- **The British Naturopathic Association is formed**, the result of a merger between the British Association of Naturopaths and the nature Cure Association of Great Britain.

- **Benedict Lust, founder of Naturopathy, dies** on September 5, 1945. For the last two years of his life, his vitality had been steadily declining, which he attributed to his being involuntarily treated with sulfa drugs. In 1943, fire broke out at one of his two "Yungborn" retreats. The Tangerine, Florida sanitarium was filled with patients and Dr. Lust repeatedly re-entered the burning building to aid in evacuation. His hair and clothes caught fire and he suffered some burns and smoke inhalation. Medical doctors treated him subsequently with intravenous antibiotics, the new and powerful sulfa drugs. While having his burns tended to and receiving oxygen, he was given either sulfonamide or sulphanilimide without his knowledge or consent. While the ill effects of these drugs would be more

common knowledge a decade later, Dr. Lust's instincts told him that there had been a residual impact on his health. But by then, discouraged by the civil war in the naturopathic profession and the loss of his sanitarium, Lust did not have the determination to rebuild his health after "those poisons were forced into my bloodstream." He was said to have neglected himself in the last year of his life[*].

More disturbing, though, was the whispered suggestion that the "fire of suspicious origin" had in fact been arson, committed by paid agents of the pseudo-medical Western group which had usurped the name of the American Naturopathic Association and diverted members to itself. Although nothing would ever be proven, there was strong suspicion on the part of Dr. Lust's followers that the fire was instigated by "the renegades".

Regardless, it was evident that the strength of the Eastern group ANA, and the traditional naturopathic movement itself, would be considerably weakened without the tireless energy of Benedict Lust.

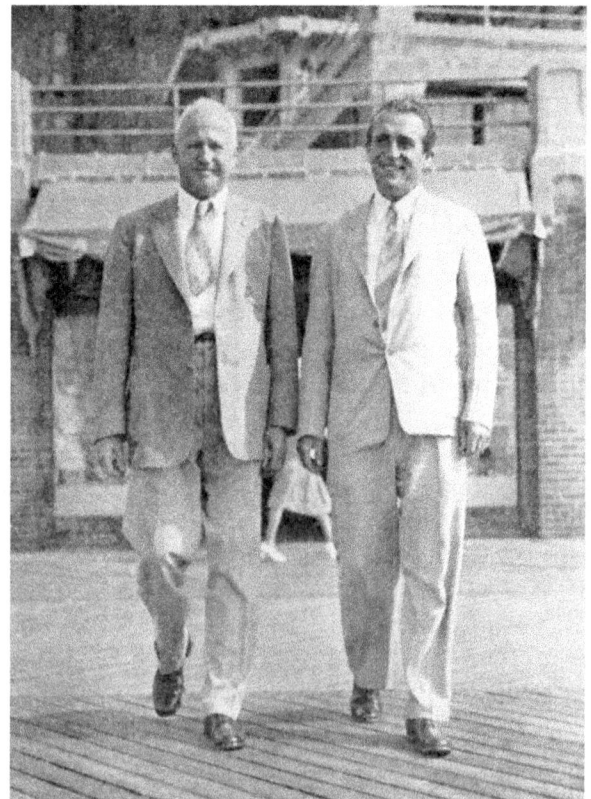

Benedict Lust outside a conference in Atlantic City with his heir apparent, Jesse Mercer Gehman.

[*] Gehman, J.M., "To Honor the Father of Naturopathy", *Nature's Path*

No other proponent of Naturopathy, with the exception of Frederick Collins, was as natural a fighter as Lust. A lifetime of battling with the medical establishment and its political machine only made him more and more determined and energetic. But in the end, it was having to do battle with his own kind that sapped the strength of the scrappy émigré from Germany who organized a whole new kind of health care. His death at 73 came earlier than most Nature Cure pioneers, and ushered in an era of increased enmity between the traditional naturopathic community and the pseudo-medical naturopathic movement.

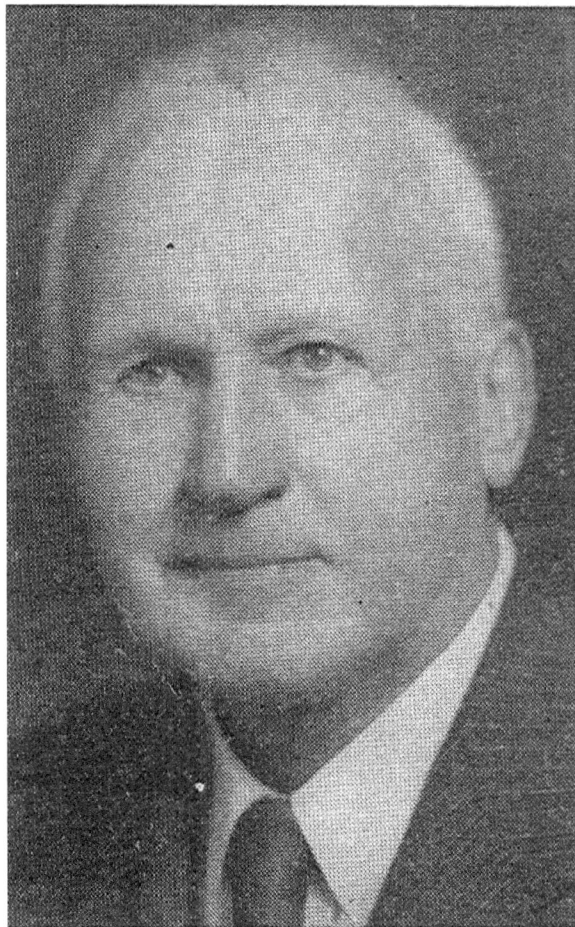

"I have been arrested 17 times, I have been handcuffed, fingerprinted, transported in the Black Maria and have slept in the Tombs for teaching and practicing the natural methods of living and healing. I was found guilty of running a school for forty years, to back up every legislative move and to safeguard the future of Naturopathy and to give the naturopathic profession a chance to earn a living, and for that I received a sentence of one year in Sing Sing. The sentence was suspended but I was stamped a criminal and if they ever get their hands on me again they will send me to jail because there can be no second suspended sentence."

--Benedict Lust

1946—

- **Two major naturopathic textbooks see print:** Thomas T. Lake, DC, ND, writes *Treatment by Neuropathy and the Encyclopedia of Physical and Manipulative Therapuetics*, and a new edition of *Principles and Practice of Drugless Therapeutics* by A.C. Johnson, DC, ND.

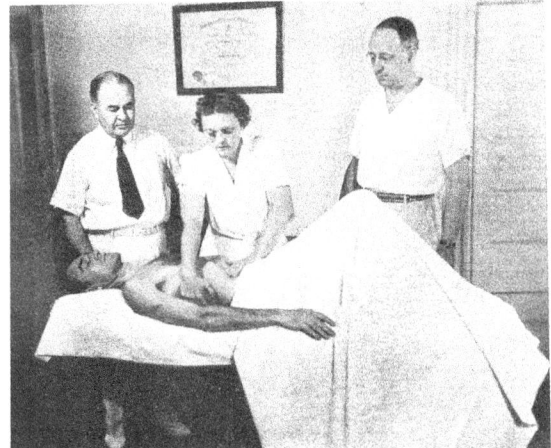

Dr. Thomas Lake looks on from the far left as visceral manipulation is applied to patient.

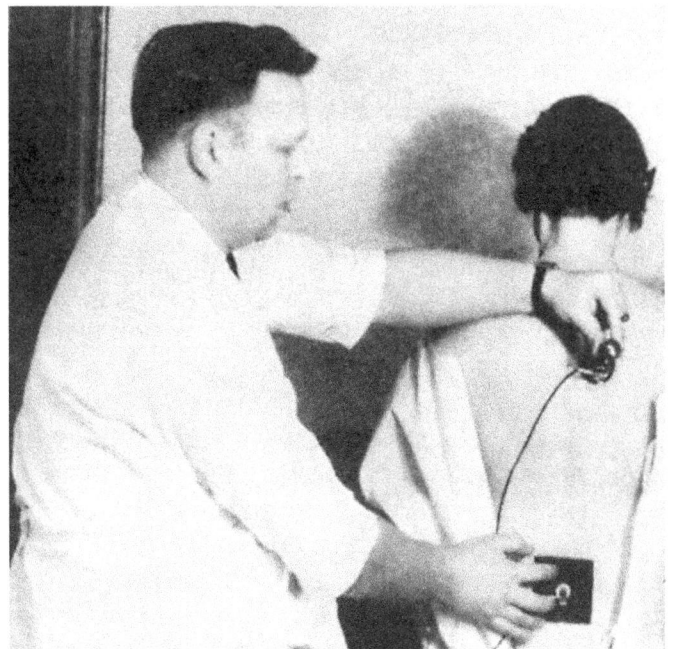

Dr. Alton C. Johnson demonstrating electrotherapy.

- A third book (but with limited circulation), *Cycle of Health*, is written by M.O. Garten, DC, ND. Garten will go on to write several popular books in the 1960s.

65

and HERALD OF HEALTH

NATUROPATH

Official Journal
of
Recognized Technicians
in
CHIROPRACTIC·PHYSIOTHERAPY·OSTEOPATHY
DIETETICS·NEUROPATHY·COSMOTHERAPY
OSMOTHERAPY·HOMEOPATHY·ECLECTICISM
and all other advanced branches of Natural Therapeutics

AMERICAN NATUROPATHIC ASSOCIATION

DR. LUST'S SOLILOQUIES

"A Merry Christmas"

Auto-Intoxication or Self-Poisoning

Should Medicine Be Socialized?

Curing Elements of Naturopathy

Thomsonian Treatment of Fevers

Massage for that Tired Feeling

Greetings to All Naturopaths

Nature Cure Is Practical

Vegetarianism—The Key

Your Doubts Dispelled

Full Index for Year of 1945

December
1945

25¢

$3.00 per year

Lesson CCXXXIX
Post Graduate Study of Naturopathy

FOUNDED 1896
BY
DR. BENEDICT LUST

VOLUME L
No. 12
CURRENT NUMBER
605

- **The United Naturopathic Physicians Association, Inc.** is formed by a group of DC/ND practitioners in California. Doctors Charles H. Wood, Floyd G. Fisk, Richard Curtis, and Frances Hammond are officers. They also publish the journal *California Naturopath.*

- **Thomas Deschauer, DC, ND, dies.** A German Nature Cure transplant, he was a noted naturopathic expert in herbalism. Living in Maywood, Illinois, Deschauer was author of several books on botanical medicine, finishing this year's new edition of the two-volume *Illustrated Phytotherapy* before his death. In 1940 he published *A Complete Course in Herbalism,* which was well-received despite a small print run. The first edition of *Illustrated Phytotherapy* was in 1942.

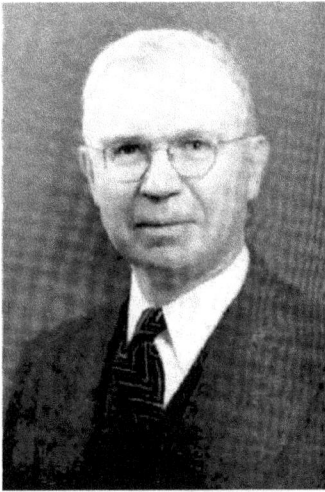

- **Sinai Gershanek, DC, ND, dies.** Benedict Lust's right-hand man in the early days of the American School of Naturopathy, he was part of the original faculty of the school. He was later head of the Metropolitan Institute of Chiropractic, also in New York City, and editor-publisher of the *Journal of Healing Arts.*

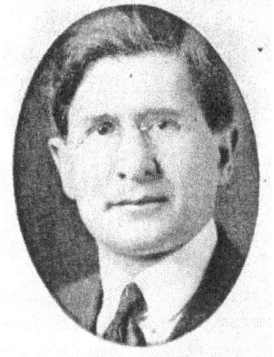

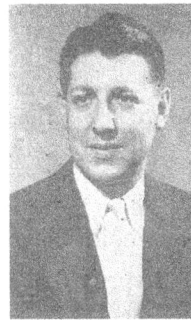

John B. Lust

- **John B. Lust**, Benedict Lust's nephew, takes over publication of the two longtime periodicals: *The Naturopath and Herald of Health* and *Nature's Path.* Lust, who earned an ND but did not practice, would author a number of health books, such as *Lust For Living,* and *The Herb Book*, an excellent reference for botanical medicines. He was the heir to the Lust legacy and would reprint his uncle's writings for decades.

- **The Naturopathic Practice Act passes in Manitoba, Canada.**

Meanwhile, across the globe…

Mahatma Ghandi visits Uruli Kanchan, a 150-bed naturopathic hospital he helped establish, in March 1946 and sees thousands of patients treated with natural methods. The hospital is under the direction of Dr. Dinshah Mehta, Dr. Sushila Mehr, and Dr. Manibhai Desai. Father of the Nation Ghandi calls for nature cure clinics to be available in all rural areas in India.

1947—

- **Tennessee repeals its naturopathic licensing law** and makes it illegal to practice Naturopathy. Licensure had only been in existence since 1943.

- **The 50th Annual Congress of the American Naturopathic Association, the "Golden Jubilee" celebration is held in New York.** Although the event is noteworthy, attendance is sparse. Rival ANA organization members of the Western group fail to attend. Because of the efforts of this splinter group to increasingly medicalize naturopathic practice, as well as split the profession, the officials of the original (Eastern) ANA felt it necessary to reiterate the traditional viewpoint of the profession, stating:

  > "Naturopathy does not make use of synthetic or inorganic vitamins or minerals, or of drugs, narcotics, surgery, serums, vaccines, anti-toxins, toxoid, injections or inoculations..."

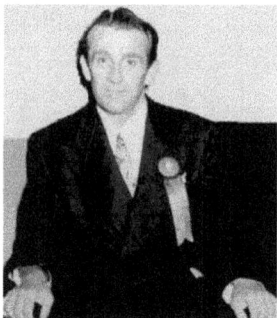

J.M. Gehman, ND

Dr. Jesse Mercer Gehman, President of the Eastern ANA, stated candidly in a bulletin shortly after the conference:

"After the miserable failure of the pseudo group to stop the Golden Jubilee...one would think that it would desist and admit its error and wrongs. But no, it continues its vicious propaganda to mislead physicians everywhere, while at the same time its officers plead they want harmony and unification. **What they want is domination...Observe their efforts**...We condemn the persistent efforts of those who know better to mislead the field." [emphasis ours]*

- **Henry Schlichting, Jr., ND**, secretary of the Western ANA and owner of the Midland (Texas) Naturopathic Clinic, joins the American Public Health Association, an organization populated mostly by medical doctors.❖ He is likely the first naturopath to apply for membership, and this unheralded event illustrates the direction the typical western ANA member was going: creating legitimacy by cultivating a public presentation as close to medical doctors as possible.

- **Dr. Charles H. Wood** of the California-based United Naturopathic Physicians Association, Inc. becomes editor of the *National Journal of the American Naturopathic Association*

OFFICERS AND MEMBERS OF THE EXECUTIVE BOARD OF THE NATUROPATHIC PHYSICIANS ASSOCIATION

Executive office of the Association:
1123 West Florence Avenue
Los Angeles, Calif.
Phone TWinoaks 3281

Dr. Paul Hunt, President — Dr. Ernest Webster, Vice President — Dr. J. W. Schmitz, Secretary — Dr. C. C. Cogill, Chairman of the Executive Board — Dr. John Heldgen, Treasurer — Dr. Geo. I. Shafer, Board Member — Dr. W. J. M. Maxwell, Board Member

- **Dr. Joe Shelby Riley dies at 90;** he introduced Zone Therapy into naturopathic practice and wrote twenty books on natural medicine, including *Great Herbal Remedies, Spinal Concussion, Reflex Technique, Remarkable Formulas,* and *Iridiagnosis.* He was the founder of the National University of Therapeutics in Washington, D.C.*

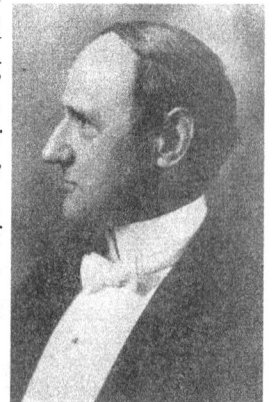

---

* "From the Office of the President: Pseudo-Group Once Again Misleading the Naturopathic Field" (Official ANA Bulletin, January 25, 1948:7-8).

❖ *Am J Pub Health,* Sept. 1947, p. 1224

* As reported in *Herald of Health and Naturopath,* July 1947

68

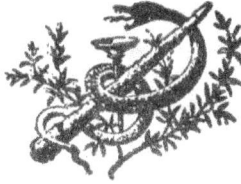

DR. FREDERICK W. COLLINS

47 SOUTH 11TH STREET
NEWARK 7, N. J.

TELEPHONES
HU. 3-4002
HU. 2-4447

August 7th, 1947.

Dr. Edward Collins,
25 E. Blackwell St.,
Dover, New Jersey.

Dear Ed,

I feel very happy today in consideration of the fact that at the Golden Jubilee Convention of the American Naturopathic Association, Inc., held at the Hotel Commodore, New York City, from July 27th to August 2nd, at the Grand Ceremonial Banquet, I was nominated to receive a certificate of award stating that I was the Master Technician of Mechanistic Therapy of the World and I was also nominated to receive a certificate of award as Dean of Naturopathy, being the last one of the five great Naturopaths of America, Lust, Lindlahr, Collins, Riley and Tilden, the other four having passed to the Great Beyond. In addition to this I was presented with a plaque. On the right side of the plaque it says:- "To F.W. Collins, N.D., in appreciation of your fifty years of service to humanity and Naturopathy" and on the left side there is a cross with the sun raying from all corners. On this plaque is written a prayer, as follows:-

A
PRAYER
Not more of light do I ask Oh
GOD!
But eyes to see what is.,
    Not sweeter songs,
But ears to hear the present Melodies,
    Not greater strength,
But how to use the Power that I possess;
    Not more of Love,
But skill to turn a frown into a caress;
    Not more of Joy,
But Power to feel its kindling presence near;
To give to others what I possess of courage and of
                                    cheer.

Give me Oh God! all fears to dominate,
    All Holy Joys to know,
To be the friend I wish to be,
    To tell the Truth I know.
"From Your Loyal Students - Naturopathic Physicians of America."

Vigorously yours,

Your loving Dad,

Frdk. W. Collins N.D..D.M.

A heartwarming letter from Frederick Collins
to his son. 1947.

1948—

- An attempted unification of the opposing factions of the American Naturopathic Association fails.

ANNOUNCEMENT

just received from the National Unification Committee

A Combined Convention of Eastern and Western Groups will be held at the Hamilton Hotel, Chicago, Illinois, on November 11th and 12th, 1949. All members of both groups are requested to reserve these dates and to be on hand to participate in this milestone event of national importance.

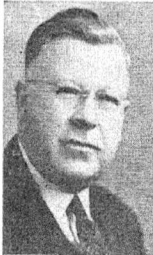

PAGE 2   JOURNAL OF THE A. N. A., INC., FOR FEBRUARY, 1948

Unification in 1948

DR. ROBERT V. CARROLL

Fellow Naturopaths:

A Happy, Joyous and Prosperous New Year to All!

A few days before Christmas we received the encouraging and splendid news that the Board of Directors of the Eastern Group had met in Washington, D. C., and voted for unity of organization. They also voted to accept our invitation to meet with us in Salt Lake City on the convention date already specified for next June.

Letters were received from Dr. Shippell and Dr. Floden, Board Chairman, notifying us of the action taken. We shall be happy to do our part in this unification program.

Dr. Floden as chairman of the one Board and Dr. Hale as chairman of the other Board will meet together soon and try to work out satisfactory methods of procedure. They will then submit their proposals to both Boards for ratification and when accepted the dark mists of past differences will be obliterated by the bright sunshine of a new day for Naturopathy.

With *unity* in the offing let us all begin to plan *now* for the coming Salt Lake City convention.

Naturopathy is not the property of any one individual or any group of individuals. Naturopathy is a definite branch of the healing arts, with sound basic principles. Let us unite and fight for those principles and there is no better time to start than *right now*. There are many things that are behind schedule on our program. We must roll up our sleeves and get deep into the work of accomplishment.

We are badly in need of a weekly publication through which we can reach the public with our side of the story. The public is looking for and seeking health. Naturopathy offers the answer. Let us tell them of the benefits to be derived through its service. We need to reach the legislatures. Our most effective way to do so is through public demand. Let the *public* tell their representatives that Naturopathy is desired and watch their positive action in its favor. With Naturopathic unity an accomplished fact, working "one for all and all for one" for Naturopathy we can and must go places. Let's make our slogan "1948 for Naturopathy."

News items from the field and articles of interest to the profession will be appreciated but no anonymous contributions will be considered.

"It is one of the most beautiful compensations of this life that no man can sincerely try to help another without helping himself."

You cannot build with safety extra rungs into your ladder of life by tearing them out of another's structure.

No pers[...] portant to [...] ily but the [...] his passing [...] in the path [...] to grow to [...] to the welf[...]

"Gold a[...] separated [...] when place [...] test. No [...] long delaye [...] ence of [...] works ye sl[...]

On the [...] where I w[...] prominentl[...] "If you sh[...] where you [...] get along w[...] call at the [...] of the gr[...] nature is a [...] our own i[...] double che[...] our own pr[...]

Rememb[...] life you m[...] you are. A [...] something [...]

If you a[...] fellow do[...] docs.

Hours ar[...] are *given* b[...] tee in orde[...] creative a[...] small bit b[...] tion and b[...]

Have yo[...] and ideas [...] fellow pr[...] will be gla[...] space your [...] side of the [...]

- **Harry Riley Spitler, N.D. of Central States College** of Physiatrics is commissioned in 1945 to write a definitive textbook for the profession. The result is 1948's *Basic Naturopathy, A Textbook*. It is published by the American Naturopathic Association.

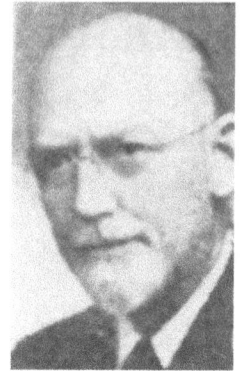

- **Adolphus Hohensee, ND runs afoul of the medical establishment** with his success. The Scranton, Pennsylvania naturopath who restored thousands of people's health through dietary means and with nutritional supplements was becoming well known from his lecture tour. Over 250,000 people had taken his courses and many more were buying the vitamins he formulated. He also established a health resort and was curing many cases of chronic disease. He found himself on trial in February 1948 in Arizona for having shipped a package of vitamins there —to *himself*—for use in an upcoming lecture. The Food and Drug Administration said that they were "misbranded" items. Although a government chemist who examined the goods when they were seized said they were "exactly according to label", by the time the trial commenced, another government witness contradicted the report of the first examiner. Ten medical doctors were brought in to testify that vitamins were not necessary in the human body. When the defense produced government bulletins claiming the opposite, the expert witnesses said they were "outdated". Dr. Hohensee was convicted and ordered to pay a fine. Moreover, the judge said that Dr. Hohensee must go to jail until the fine was paid, and denied his right to appeal the case.

1948—

- The Western ANA organization begins publication of the *Journal of the American Naturopathic Association* in January 1948. Initial issues feature the familiar ANA symbol used for years by the Eastern group…

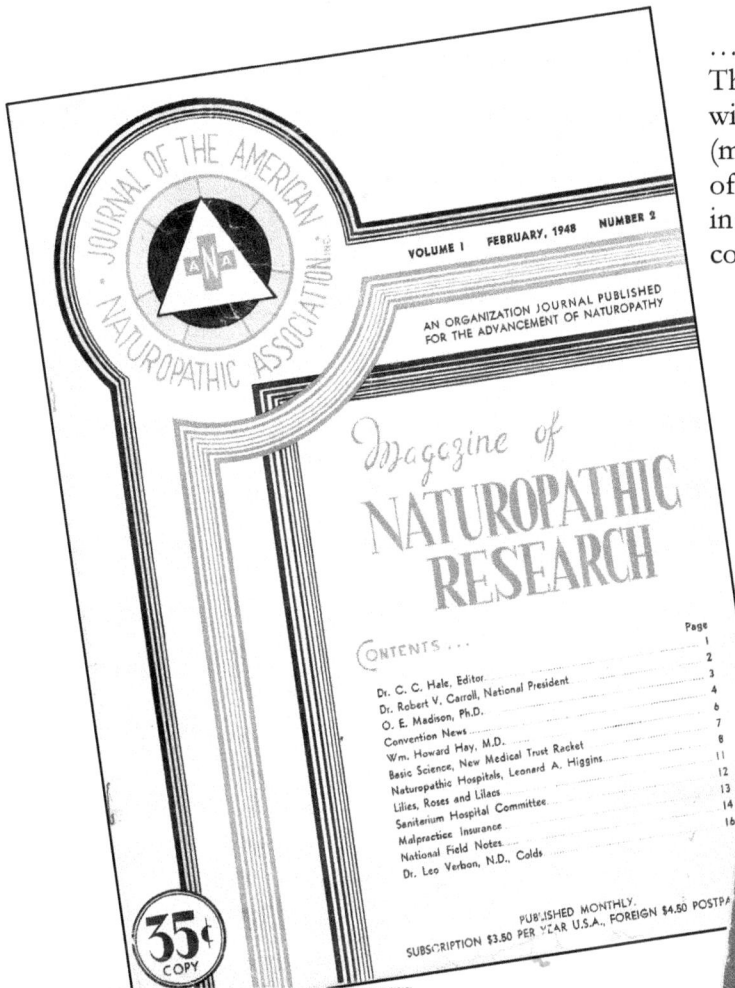

…by the next year, however, it bears a new logo. There was clearly not even a pretense of fraternity with the original organization any longer. This symbol (more conforming to the usual medical *caduceus*) would often appear, with some variations, in the years ahead in the increasingly pseudo-medical naturopathic community.

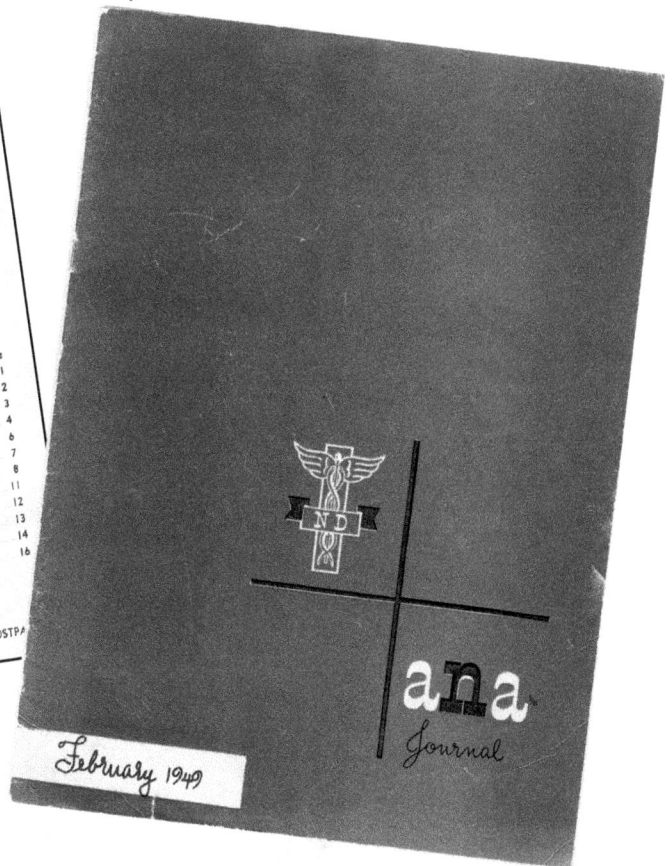

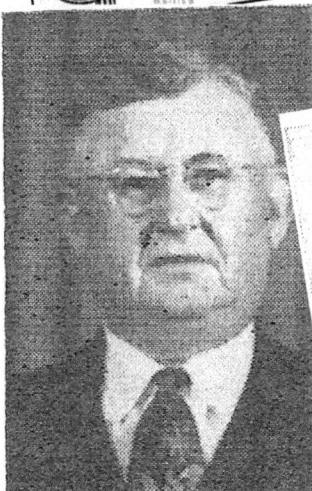

Henry Schlichting, Sr., ND

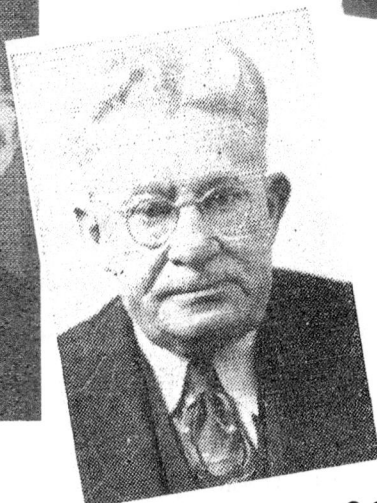

C.C. Hale, ND

HERALD of HEALTH
and Naturopath

Associate Departments in
CHIROPRACTIC · PHYSIOTHERAPY · OSTEOPATHY
and all other Branches of Natural Therapeutics

FOUNDED 1896
BY
Dr. BENEDICT LUST

AUGUST
1948

20¢

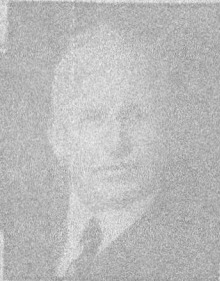

This Month With Dr. Schippell
"Naturopathy — and Time"

The Doctors Talk It Over
"Thumbs Down"

Dr. Lust Speaking
"The Good and the Bad"

**Gaining Weight is Really a Matter
of Gaining Health**
Gayelord Hauser

"The Paradox of Death"
Philip Friedman

California — and the Thirty Pieces of Silver
Dr. T. M. Schippell

Arthritis — Its Cause and Cure
Dr. Richard A. Lynch

The True Naturopath Seeks a Cure
Dr. Frank E. Dorchester

When You Are Sick Blame Yourself
Dr. Sanford B. Manks

Are Your Cosmetics Dangerous Poisons?
Benjamin D. Baxter

Home Study Course
in Naturopathy

Book Reviews
Reader's Column

Current No. 636

Volume 53   NOW - $2.00 per Year - ANYWHERE !   Number 8

Dr. Lust's monthly magazine would continue in his absence, however--with his regular column intact, as though he was still watching over his flock, the original ANA.

1948—(cont.)

- **Los Angeles College of Chiropractic stops awarding naturopathic degrees** and discontinues herbology courses in the wake of strong opposition to "liberal" or "mixer" practice of Chiropractic.

- **Cleveland's Metropolitan College ceases operations.** Their registry and alumni are transferred to National College in Chicago.

- **Dr. Frederick W. Collins dies.** He was the founder of First National University and United States School of Naturopathy. He was considered by many to be the greatest contributor to the field after Benedict Lust, and in fact was Lust's favored candidate for successor. Due to Collins' fighting for Naturopathy in court, the Supreme Court of New Jersey handed down twenty-five decisions favorable to natural medicine[*]. The Court of Appeals confirmed, among other things, that naturopaths were not to be judged by the standards of any other school of medicine (this was at a time when states were using "basic science" legislation to exclude from practice those who did not attend allopathic schools). He was the last of the original "big five" naturopathic pioneers in the U.S.--outliving Lust, Lindlahr, Tilden, and Riley.

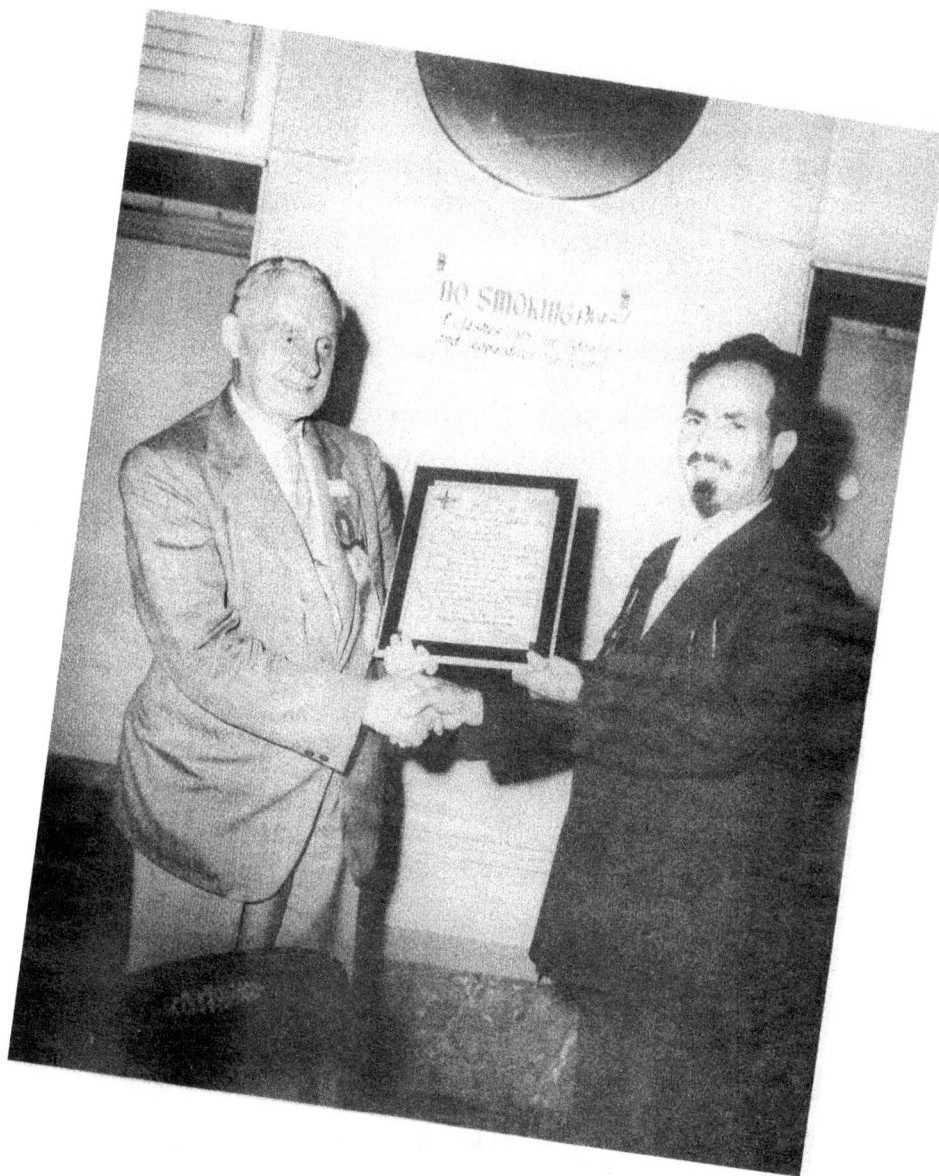

Dr. Collins (left) receives award from Dr. Eppolito of New York in appreciation from the naturopathic profession.

---

[*] Collins v. Tansey

73

1948—

- Robert Carroll's brother, famed naturopath **Otis Carroll, attended the conventions of both factions of the ANA** in 1947. He later spoke before the original American Naturopathic Association gathering in New York, and made this prediction, which in light of the events to come in the 1980s, is remarkable:

> "You are either all going to get together or you are lost. I want to warn you that when I attended the convention in Detroit, I found the best group of high pressure salesmen that any group has. They have all withdrawn from us [the Eastern ANA]. They don't argue with me, but I am a brother of the president of that association, and there is no better high pressure salesman than he is. He has a sales group of men around him who are just as good as he is and **they are going to overcome you…Remember, that group of people are pseudo medical men and just as soon as they get power they are going to be no better."**
>
> --O. G. Carroll, ND

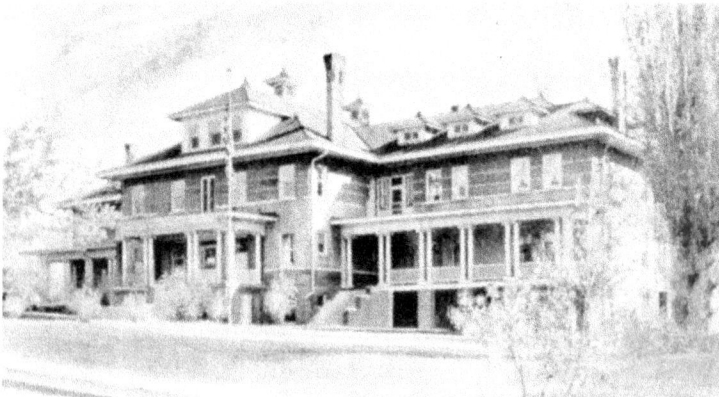

1949—

- **Mario Campanella, ND**, of Graham, Florida, is elected president of the International Society of Naturopathic Physicians.

- **Joint convention** is held between the International Society of Naturopathic Physicians and the American Naturopathic Association. Past President of ISNP Dr. Arthur Schramm begs again for unification of Eastern and Western ANA organizations. [*]

- **Texas licenses naturopathic doctors.**

- The **British College of Naturopathy** is founded.

- **A convention is scheduled for November in Chicago that would supposedly unite Eastern and Western factions of the ANA.** This is arranged by the Western ANA. Jesse Mercer Gehman, president of the Eastern ANA, says their board refuses to participate.

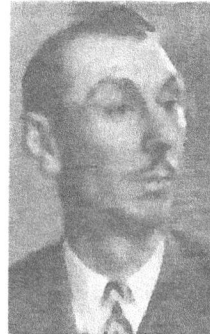

Schlichting

The convention is cancelled. The following month, Western ANA president Henry Schlichting Jr. wrote in an editorial about unification of the two groups that "…I believe this was also in agreement with the wishes of the vast majority of the profession."[♦]

- **American Naturopathic Hospital** is established in Salt Lake City in 1949 to serve as a clinical training facility. This was formerly the Pyott Sanitarium, a private naturopathic institution[•].

[*] *Journal of the American Naturopathic Association, Inc.*, Oct. 1949, p. 17

[♦] *Journal of the American Naturopathic Association*, October 1949

[•] *Journal of the American Naturopathic Association*, June 1949

1949—

- **Naturopaths using their unconventional methods still continue to draw the ire of the orthodox medical community.** Methods are often attacked in proportion to their effectiveness. Those that are opposed the most strongly were often the most reliable for conditions that are ordinarily thought to be resolved only by drugs and surgery. In this way, natural medicine was diverting many dollars from local hospitals and this did not go unnoticed.

While the use of proprietary supplements or specific herbs, etc., could be pronounced "dangerous" and access to them blocked, it was difficult to interfere with those therapies that did not use exotic substances or manufactured goods. It was next to impossible to cut off a naturopath's access to whole foods, water, or light. But in this last example—the use of concentrated light as a therapy—equipment *was* manufactured and used by the profession. The use of light in the visible spectrum was embraced by the naturopathic profession, and the producers of equipment for that practice felt the wrath of the Food and Drug Administration. This photo from the Milwaukee Journal, Oct. 15, 1949, shows thirty light therapy machines confiscated from natural medicine practices and being destroyed by government agents as "fake healing machines".

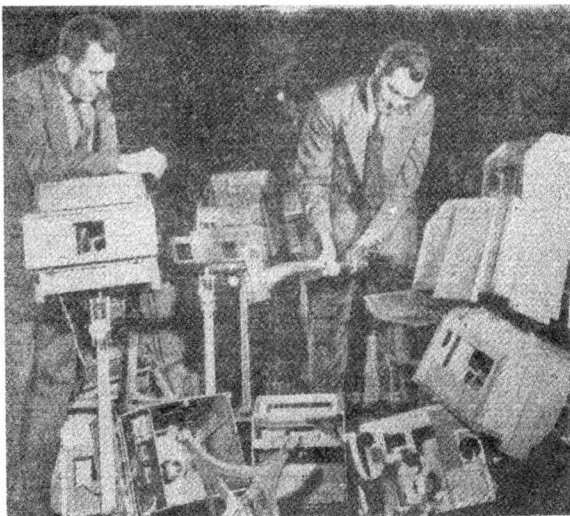

- **A bill to repeal the Naturopathic Licensing law was introduced into the Florida legislature.** The following newspaper article gives the picture:

PENSACOLA (Florida) JOURNAL, April 15, 1949

NATUROPATHS' USE OF DRUGS TERMED 'DANGEROUS' BY SOWDER

Jacksonville (Special)—The state board of health has information indicating that Naturopathy as is now being practiced may be "dangerous" to the public health, Dr. Wilson T Sowder, state health officer, declared Thursday.

His statement followed a recommendation by the state board of health to the legislature that the practice of Naturopathy be investigated and if found to be detrimental to the public health, that proper legislation be enacted to correct the evils found.

Dr. Sowder gave the following information as the basis for the board's recommendations:

"The licensing board for Naturopaths was set up with the understanding that their practice would be carried on without using drugs or surgery—that natural methods of healing be used, such as diet, sunshine, fresh air, exercise, employment of hot and cold water.

Drugless Physicians

"Another name for Naturopathy is drugless physicians. At the time the licensure law was passed for Naturopaths, they were supposed to be against the use of drugs, stating that drugs were poisonous. They were also against the use of serums, such as smallpox vaccine. According to their journals, they did not believe germs caused diseases.

"However, the practitioners of this art evidently have changed their minds and now say that they cannot carry on their practice without the use of morphine, the strongest, and its derivatives.

"The state board of health is opposed to Naturopaths using drugs because it is believed they have not had training in the use of drugs. The Federal Bureau of Narcotics has also expressed concern about this."

Dr. Sowder pointed out that Florida is the only state where Naturopaths are permitted the use of drugs.

(Continued next page)

(Cont.)

The Tennessee legislature recently investigated and subsequently withdrew the licenses of approximately 1,000 Naturopaths. Out of that group, 66 are now in practice in Florida.

Another reason for the state board of health's concern is that it is difficult for the average person to distinguish between offices of Naturopaths and those of other practitioners," he said. "Naturopaths use signs such as 'Dr. John Doe', and although the law requires that the branch of healing art be shown, this is abbreviated and the sign placed in an inconvenient place," he added.

Senator Philip D. Beal of Pensacola has introduced a bill with a view to correct the situation."

1950—

- The Western faction of the American Naturopathic Association claims that both Eastern and Western groups merged into a new organization, the **American Naturopathic Physicians and Surgeons Association**. The Eastern "parent body" ANA denies such a merger and continues operating independently.[*]

An anonymous writer, putting a paid advertisement in the journal *American Naturopath* a few years later, expressed his views, which he or she must have felt might be suppressed otherwise:

"The national naturopathic organization picture has had varied experiences of storm and staleness—and after what I hear—with very little in between. As I understand it, the weakness is equal among our three known national organizations. Only a very few years ago, when the latest such national formation took place, that newest addition was sneeringly called "renegade" with willing predictions of doom. This, in a little while of course, seemed almost justifiable in view of the ridiculous top-heavy salary they obligated themselves for—to pay to certain individual[s]."

[*] *Journal of Naturopathic Medicine*, Sept. 1950, p. 20

76

Send Students

to the Naturopathic Schools and Colleges approved by the A.N.A. Council on Schools and Colleges:

CLASS A

Central States College, Eaton, Ohio

Western States College, Portland, Oregon

Arizona College of Naturopathic Medicine, Bisbee, Arizona (Re-opening September 1, 1949

APPROVED:

Texas College of Naturopathy, Dallas, Texas, Resident Course

American Therapy College, Ironton, Missouri, Resident Course

- **Georgia licenses naturopathic doctors.**

- **Thomas Lake, DC, ND, dies.** He was the author of *Treatment by Neuropathy and the Encyclopedia of Physical and Manipulative Therapeutics, Endo-nasal Technic,* and *Treatment of the Prostate by Physical and Manipulative Therapy.*

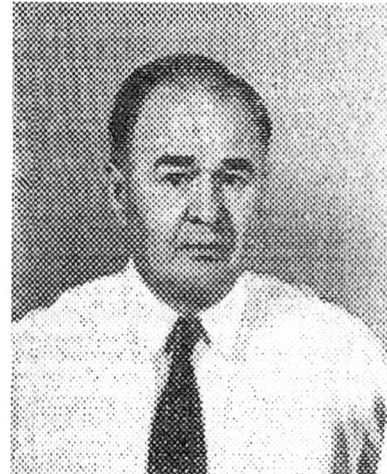

Thomas Lake, DC, ND

Nature's Path

Health through Rational Living

APRIL-1950
25c (IN CANADA 35c)

AMERICA'S PIONEER HEALTH MAGAZINE·FOUNDED IN 1896·BY DR. BENEDICT LUST·

MODERN PHYSIOTHERAPY IN ARTHRITIS

BY H. WM. BAUM, N.D.

No age is immune to Arthritis. There are at least twenty distinct types under the two headings, "rheumatoid" or "osteo."

Physiotherapy provides those physical measures that have been used for treatment since ancient times developed to the perfection of a science. The tone of despair in the sufferer's voice when he says "I have Arthritis" is changed to a note of confidence by Dr. Baum.

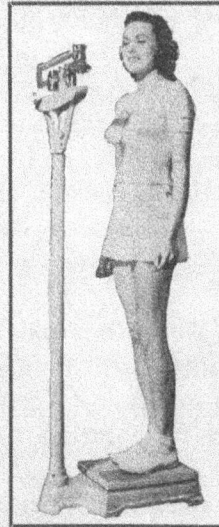

APPENDICITIS
BY DR. WM. R. LUCAS

THE NERVOUS BREAKDOWN
BY DR. ALICE CHASE

VITAMIN FACTORS IN DIET THERAPY
BY DR. W. F. WRATTEN

ENDOCRINE GLANDS
BY DR. JUAN AMON-WILKINS

ORGANIC FOODS
BY DR. JACOB H. MILLER

**HEALTH PROBLEMS • HOBBIES • MENUS
ALL FOR A WHOLESOME, HAPPY LIFE**

AMERICA'S OLDEST, LARGEST, AND MOST MODERN NATURAL HEALTH MAGAZINE   ESTABLISHED IN 1896

While *Herald of Health and Naturopath* was the publication for practitioners, *Nature's Path* was the magazine published by the eastern ANA to reach the public. Also established by Benedict Lust, it was published regularly for decades.

1951—

- **Dr. Paul Wendel's** *Standardized Naturopathy* **textbook is published.**[*] It provides a picture of the profession at this time and gives voice to the more traditional approach at a time when the pseudo-medical version of Naturopathy was growing.

- **Bernard Jensen, DC, ND** writes *The Science and Practice of Irididology.*

- **Naturopathic Institute of Los Angeles,** founded in 1909 by Carl Schultz, ND, closes.

- **Robert V. Carroll, ND dies.** He was one of the chief architects of the new pseudo-medical naturopathic profession. His son Bobby, also a naturopath, will take his place among the newer generation of modern naturopathic organizers.

- **In Arizona, A.W. Kuts-Cheraux, ND, filed suit against the State Attorney General**[*] to counter the repeated prosecutions of naturopaths there for practicing medicine without a license. The issue was the administering of natural medicines, which the court held was not within the scope of practice of a naturopath, since the law used the phrase "...excepting material medica and major surgery". As naturopaths were licensed as "drugless healers", the right to prescribe was denied. Kuts-Cheraux would later write *Naturae Medicina*, a guide to botanical medicines, in another two years.

1952—

- **Southern College of Naturopathic Medicine** in Brownsville, Texas closes its doors.

- **Naturopathic Practice Act becomes law in Alberta, Canada.**

- **W. Martin Bleything, N.D.** wrote in the July 1952 edition of the Journal of the ANPSA:

"...Thus was born the monster of faction which had so successfully prevented advancement in the past. This monster continued to grow in ferocity if not in stature until about two years ago when the two leading groups met in St. Louis and amalgamated into the present American Naturopathic Physicians and Surgeons Association.

"Although there were a few diehards who contended that the amalgamation did not take place and who denied the accomplishment of amalgamation with all the vigor displayed in the past, the newly combined membership of the two groups sat in perfect order and elected officers and trustees and adopted a new constitution."

And, in a statement that is strangely prophetic when viewed from the 21st Century, Bleything comments on the accomplishments of the organization:

"The improvement in various state laws, the raising of school standards, the class of students being attracted to the profession, **the almost complete stamping out of factions and cultisms and the improved social standing of the members** [our emphasis] is evidence enough to cause any logical person to join; this is to say nothing about the advantages in strength of union and planned procedure."

Bleything would later co-found National College of Naturopathic Medicine, the first of the unapologetically "pseudo-medical" naturopathic schools.

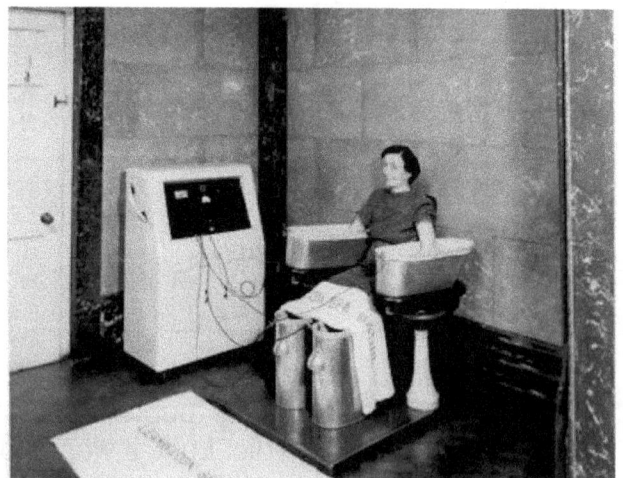

Schnee four-cell electrogalvanic bath in the early '50s

[*] Kuts-Cheraux v. Wilson, 71 Ariz. 461 (1951)

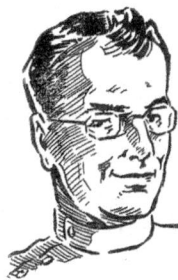

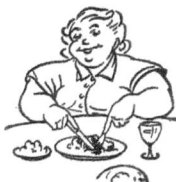

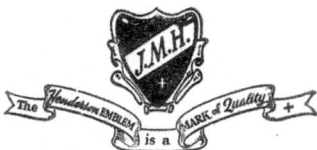

1953—

- **John R. Christopher, MH, ND opens the School of Natural Healing** in Springville, Utah. Christopher's goal was to have someone in every family trained in herbal medicine, and a practitioner in every community. By training lay people, he parted company with the naturopathic community that was struggling

for legitimacy and acceptance of its educational standards.

- *Naturae Medicina* **by A.W. Kuts-Cheraux, ND is published** by the ANPSA. It becomes the reference work for botanical medicine and the basis for naturopathic formularies in states where NDs could prescribe natural medicines.

Just as they employed herbal medicines from early in the development of the profession, naturopaths later embraced homeopathic medicines. Although he was educated in a homeopathic medical college, Benedict Lust did not emphasize the use of these natural medicines. But since their benign nature fit with the gentle, natural methodologies of Naturopathy, homeopathic remedies became part of many NDs' practices over time. This increased somewhat in proportion to the decline of homeopathic medical doctors. Homeopathic medical schools granting the MD degree had largely passed out of existence by the 1950s. Hahnemann Medical School of Philadelphia retained its homeopathic courses as electives (this would finally end in 1960). As the older practitioners were retiring or dying off, naturopaths felt impelled to rescue another natural method from disappearing. Although giving little tablets by mouth was too "medical" for some nature cureists, others went full force into the field. Always a fascinating study, Homeopathy became a common modality within the practice of Naturopathy, which was after all the most eclectic branch of the healing art. Homeopathic courses became included in the remaining naturopathic schools, and the homeopathic pharmaceutical companies also supplied naturopaths with a good supply of botanical products and other sundry items.

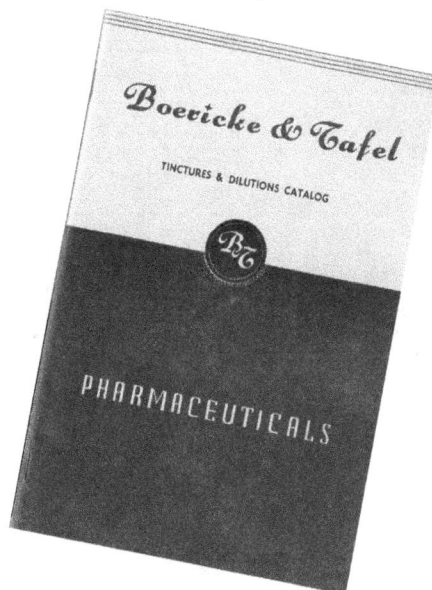

An increasing number of products were available that would today be categorized as "nutraceuticals"—materials that were made from nutritional elements but were administered for specific types of ailments. Because there were few retail outlets carrying such products, the naturopathic doctor was able to supply his or her patients with all that was needed, or refer them to the companies that sold them.

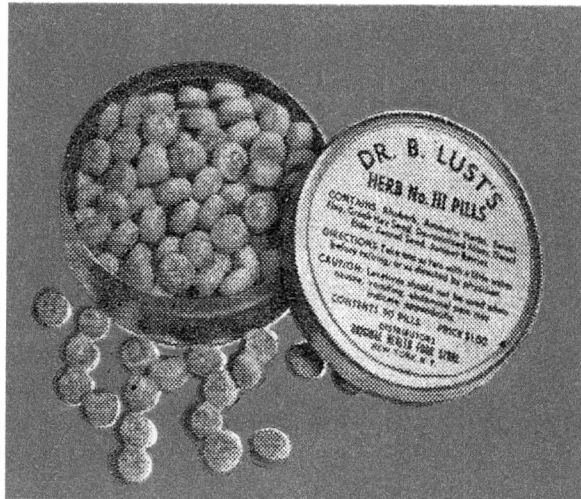

Of course, for decades one of Dr. Lust's recommended remedies had been available, and would continue to be sold long after his time. His "Herb No. 3 Pills" were a compound of laxative plant ingredients to aid detoxification of the colon.

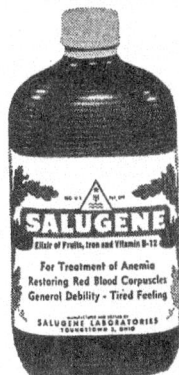

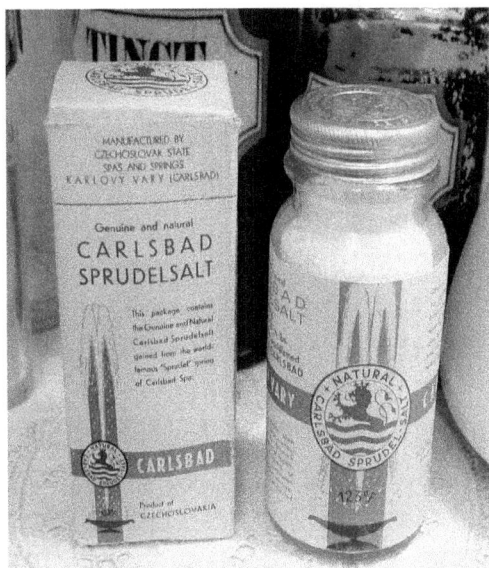

Frederick Collins did something similar with spinal manipulation and created what he variously called the *Naturopathic Tonic Treatment* or the *Collins Universal Tonic Technic*. It was a manual method that systematically freed all the articulations of the spinal segments and the rib attachments, initiated lymphatic drainage, and stimulated the organs of the abdominal cavity—all in five minutes. It could be used as part of a treatment plan for any condition—in a word, *universal*.

"Bloodless Surgery" was a method that came to the U.S. in the person of the German doctor **Adolph Lorenz**, and spread among naturopaths and chiropractors. **Joe Shelby Riley** and **Paul Wendell** headed the list of naturopaths who were well known for their prowess in this method. Wendell wrote a book on the technique that is still in print. A soft tissue manipulation that affects nerves and connective tissue, Bloodless Surgery was re-worked by the English naturopath **Stanley Leif**. By applying static deep pressure, often with a handheld tool, he went one step forward and created what he termed "Neuromuscular Technique", or NMT.

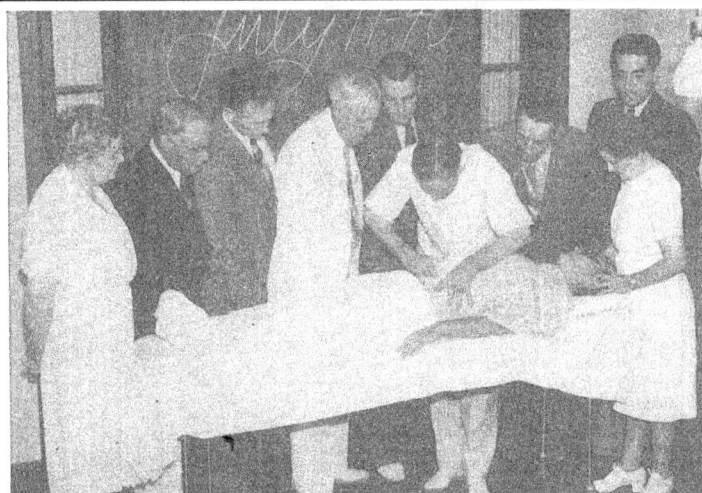

Dr. James McGinnis demonstrates during a training session in bloodless surgery.

Despite the increased dispensing of oral remedies on the part of naturopaths, there were those who kept developing and improving the low-tech methods that had been in use since the profession's infancy.

As mentioned, **O.G. Carroll** created what he termed *Constitutional Hydrotherapy* as a more efficient way to apply the most often-used water application procedures in an office setting. Because it created a systemic reaction and produced powerful effects in a short time, it could be applied to almost any condition.

Another time-tested therapy that does not rely on oral medications is *hyperthermia*. Heating of the body in a way that creates artificial fever has systemic effects that are applicable in many chronic as well as acute diseases. The light cabinet, the Schlenz bath, the Russian bath and the fever cabinet have all been used to harness the terrific power of fever to cure illness. An interesting device to achieve this was the Therm-Aire apparatus, an air mattress with a heating coil inside and a heated blanket over it. The patient is slowly heated while cooling air is directed to the head.

Chloe Ruth Jay, ND monitors the patient's vital signs in the picture below. Dr. Jay's practice was focused on detoxification through hyperthermia.

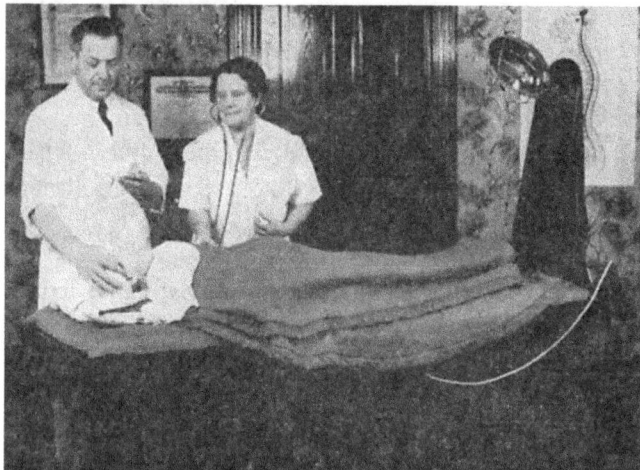

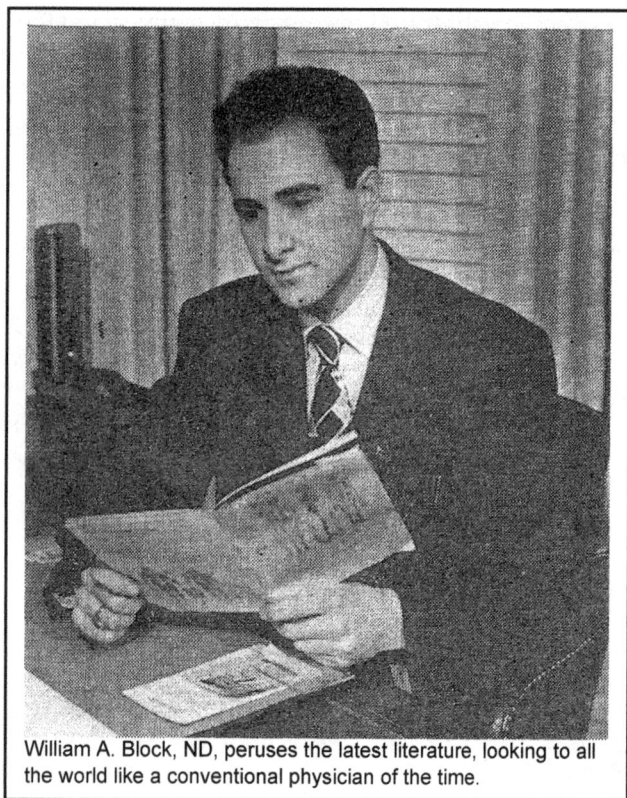
William A. Block, ND, peruses the latest literature, looking to all the world like a conventional physician of the time.

1954—

- A Naturopathic Practice Act becomes law in Saskatchewan, Canada.

- The American Naturopathic Physicians and Surgeons Association changes its name to **American Association of Naturopathic Physicians** (AANP).

A major event in naturopathic jurisprudence occurred in 1954.

The pseudo-medical naturopathic community had been using its influence to restrict licensure to its own members in several states, inducing the boards to grant the right to practice to only those whose diplomas passed one particular credentialing body. Although educational councils had been set up for years and there was more than one credentialing agency for the profession, there was now a call for one exclusive pathway to licensure.

This would be challenged by Paul Wendell, ND, President of the eastern ANA. Filing a lawsuit against the restrictive practice, he fought it to the U.S. Court of Appeals and won.

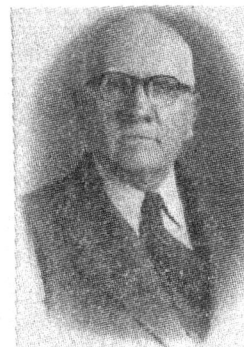
Paul Wendel, ND

This resulted in a ruling that licensing boards must accept credentials from more than one association recognizing naturopathic medicine diplomas and credentialing.

(Paul Wendell v. Samuel Spencer, the US Court of Appeals, Circuit of the District of Columbia Case #1179 *)

* Printed in the Federal Reporter #217, 2nd series, pp. 858-860

- **The National Chiropractic Association refuses accreditation to schools that also have naturopathic programs**, causing many of the remaining naturopathic educational institutions to disappear.[*]

The Los Angeles College of Chiropractic was the end result of several moves, name changes, and amalgamations of naturopathic and chiropractic schools over the years. Dr. Keating of the LACC noted that between 1922 and 1947 every president of each of the schools which ultimately became LACC held both a DC and ND degree. Seventeen out of eighteen other administrators also held both DC and ND degrees, as did nineteen of twenty-seven faculty members. But by 1947, there were six full-time professors at LACC and only five had an ND degree.

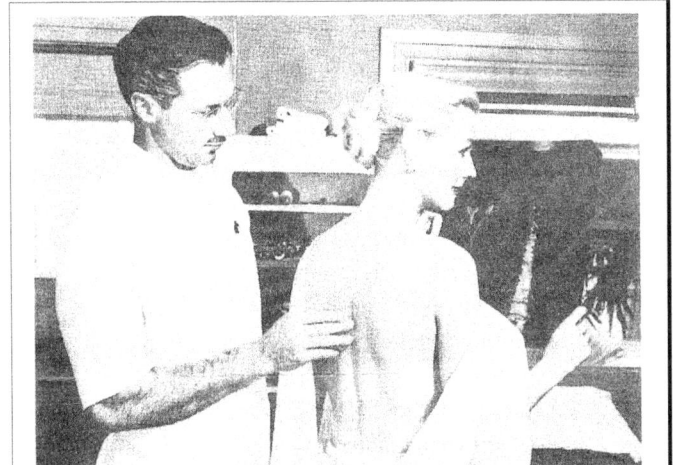

A DC/ND shows his patient her X-ray in this illustration of the profession at that time.

D.C., N.D.

The most common exponent of the natural medicine field in these days was the DC/ND practitioner. Thousands of chiropractors took extra training in natural therapeutics and became the backbone of the profession. Many chiropractic colleges with naturopathic programs had better facilities by the early 1950s than the independent naturopathic schools, and their graduates were capable practitioners. But the chiropractic field was always attacked from without and contentious within. The inclusion of naturopathic curricula became a liability, and the DC/ND became an endangered species.

[*] Holly J. Hough et al., Profile of a Profession: Naturopathic Practice, Center for the Health Professions, University of California, San Francisco, 2001

- **In Texas, the Attorney General declared the 1949 statute legalizing Naturopathy to be unconstitutional.** This 1955 reversal effectively removed the license of **Harry Hoxsey, ND**, without which he could not continue to operate his clinic, the most successful cancer treatment facility in the country at the time.

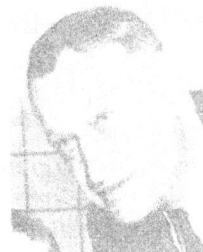

Harry Hoxsey, ND

Hoxsey received his ND from the Southern College of Naturopathy, which was also effectively put out of business a few years earlier. Hoxsey was a colorful figure with an independent income from oil wells, which allowed him to expand in a way that no naturopath ever had the luxury of doing. He used botanical medicines to treat various types of cancer; escharotics for those tumors on or close to the surface of the body, and the internal formula that was handed down to him by his father. He was persecuted by the American Medical Association and eventually won against them in court, with the AMA admitting that the Hoxsey herbal formulas did in fact cure cancers—a legal victory for natural medicine that has never been equalled.

At the peak of his activities, Hoxsey had clinics in seventeen states and no one was ever turned away for inability to pay. Constant interference and widespread negative press caused the closing of all the stateside clinics and the method has been only available in Mexico since then. Hoxsey is remembered to this day as a prime example of someone widely branded as a "quack" purely because he so effectively challenged the status quo.

- **The Australian Natural therapies Association is formed** from an amalgamation of the National Association of Naturopaths and the Australian Chiropractic, Osteopathic, and Naturopathic Physicians Association.

- **Western States College (Portland) drops its naturopathic program** and becomes chiropractic-only. Western States was a flagship naturopathic school in the Pacific Northwest, and many of the future leaders of the profession received their training there.

- **University of Healing Arts, Denver, Colorado, closes.** It had provided naturopathic education since 1934.

- **The State of Georgia eliminates the Naturopathic Board of Examiners.**

- **The State of Tennessee** makes the practice of Naturopathy a "gross misdemeanor" under the law.

- **The American Association of Naturopathic Physicians (AANP) changes its name to** *National* **Association of Naturopathic Physicians (NANP).** John W. Noble is President, John Bastyr is Vice-President. When viewed from a standpoint of many years later, the incessant name-switching during the course of only a decade seems bizarre. But it points up the tendencies in policy and decision-making among those who would demand that their vision of the modern naturopathic physician become institutionalized.◆

In the February 1956 issue of *American Naturopath*, the "independent national professional naturopathic journal", editor Carl Hotchkiss, ND says:

"To our knowledge there are at least three national naturopathic organizations and numerous state organizations—each one of which publishes its own *"official"* bulletin, journal, or other named publication…Our independent status has secured us a highly favored position as a paid subscription journal among officers and members of both national and state organizations, as well as a great number of doctors with no professional affiliation."

The monthly digest-sized journal was a readable and practical publication, with none of the political bias of other periodicals. "Our pages are free of prejudice," one blurb claimed.

Dr. Hotchkiss mused: "Have we as a profession lost the vision?"

◆ Holly J. Hough et al., *Profile of a Profession: Naturopathic Practice*, Center for the Health Professions, University of California, San Francisco, 2001

1955—

- **Max Warmbrand, ND, DO authors Add Years To Your Heart**, a popular health book introducing the public to natural methods at a time when awareness of heart disease was just beginning to grow, due to the heart attack of then-President Eisenhower.

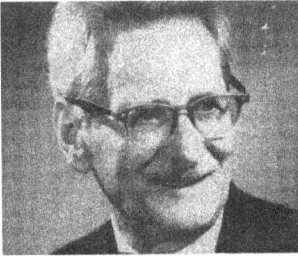

Max Warmbrand, ND, DO

1956—

- **National College of Naturopathic Medicine is founded in Portland, Oregon** by Frank Spaulding, John Bastyr, Martin Bleything and Charles Stone*. Spaulding toured the country seeking out donations from established naturopaths to start the school, insuring that the profession—and its state licenses—would not disappear. The patrons made monthly installments toward establishing the school. Spaulding collected over $100,000 in all.

1957—

- **Washington State changes its license** from "Drugless Healing" to "Naturopathic" license.

- What would later become known as the **Clymer Clinic is founded in Quakertown, Pennsylvania** by R. Swiburne Clymer, MD. As a clinic with diagnostic and treatment capabilities and completely devoted to natural medicine, this facility will influence many private naturopathic clinics in the years to come.

* Kirchfeld, Friedhelm, and Boyle, Wade. *Nature Doctors: Pioneers in Naturopathic Medicine*. Medicina Biologica, 1994

- **The State of Florida "sunsets" the naturopathic law.** The ND license is abolished after a court decision construed that the practice act—as worded—authorized naturopaths to prescribe drugs, including narcotics. While allowing those already licensed to continue practicing, the scope of practice was limited after this legislative session.

- **Dr. Adolphus Hohensee** is again brought to trial for his success in spreading the natural food movement and distributing nutritional supplements. In 1948 he had been in U.S. District Court in Arizona for shipping vitamins —to himself. Now he was arrested for having shipped ten pounds of whole wheat from Scranton, Pennsylvania to Denver, Colorado. The prosecution claimed that since Hohensee claimed health benefits for natural foods, the wheat was a "misbranded drug". Government witnesses said he shipped the wheat "without adequate directions for its use, and failed to state the purpose and conditions and diseases for which it was intended." A verdict of guilty was rendered, and the naturopath was given a sentence of year and a day in a Federal penitentiary. His wife and brother-in-law were also arrested and confined for several months and Hohensee's farm and office were ransacked for records of his satisfied clients, numbering in the hundreds of thousands.

Meanwhile, elsewhere...
- **In East Germany, the government reinstates training of heilpraktikers (naturopaths).** Training and licensure of additional naturopaths had been banned since 1949.

1958—

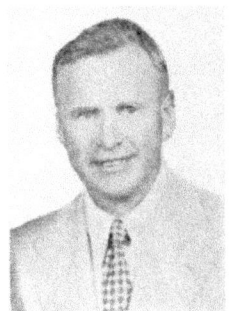

- **Max Otto Garten, DC, ND**, writes *Dynamics of Vibrant Health*, a book for the lay public that is nonetheless a solid textbook of naturopathic healing methods.

1959—

- **National College of Naturopathic Medicine relocates** to Seattle, Washington from Portland, Oregon.

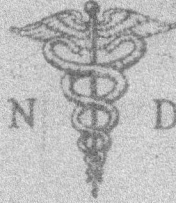

Naturopathic Physician's Oath

I swear before God and those assembled witnesses, that I will keep this oath and stipulations; to esteem those who taught me this natural healing art; to follow the method of treatment which according to my ability and judgement I consider for the benefit of my patients; to abstain from whatever is deleterious and mischievous.

With purity I will pass my life and practice my art. I will at all times consider the patients under my care as of supreme importance. I will not spare myself in rendering them the help which I have been taught to give by my Alma Mater.

Whatever in connection with my professional practice or not in connection with it I may see or hear in the lives of men and women which ought not to be spoken abroad, I will not divulge, reckoning that all such should be kept secret.

While I continue to keep this oath unviolated, may it be granted to me to enjoy life and the practice of the natural healing art respected by all men at all times. So help me God.

Naturopathic oath from the 1950s

5

DECLINE
AND
REBIRTH

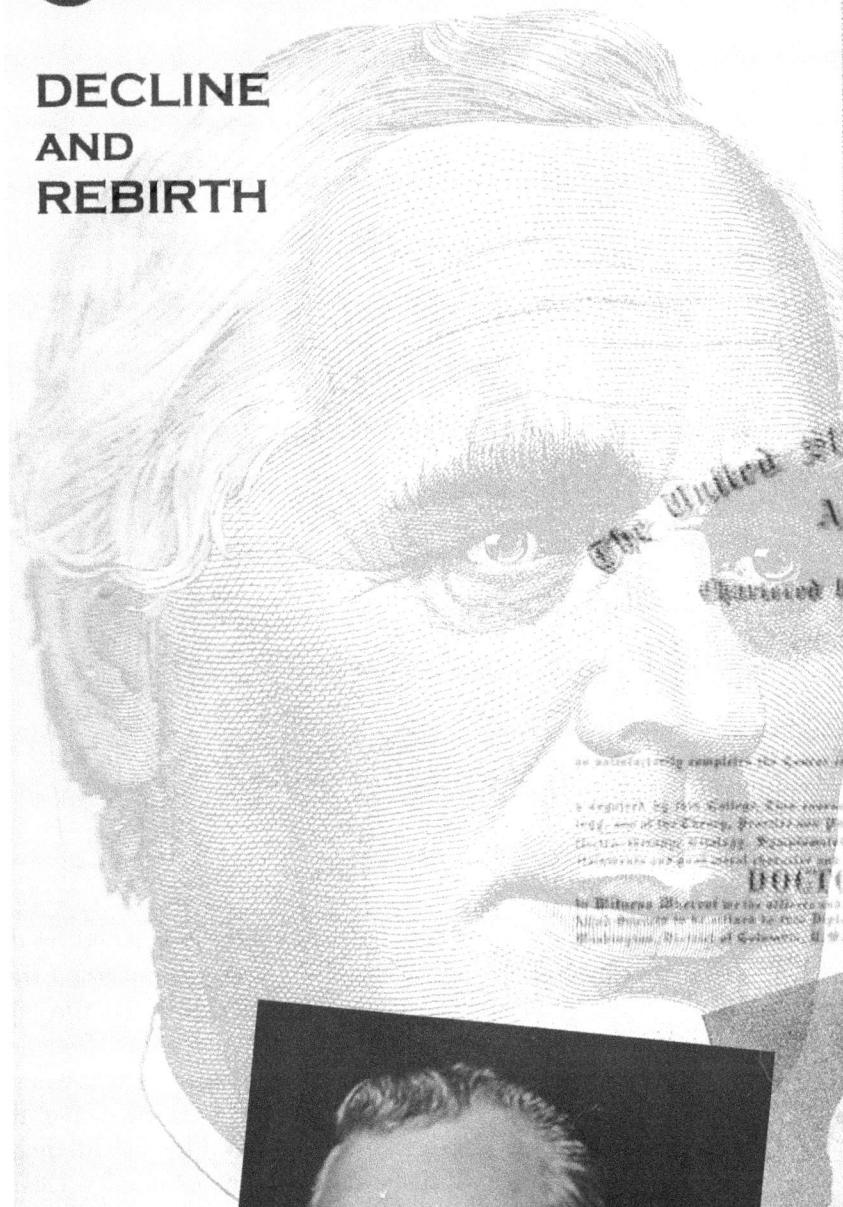

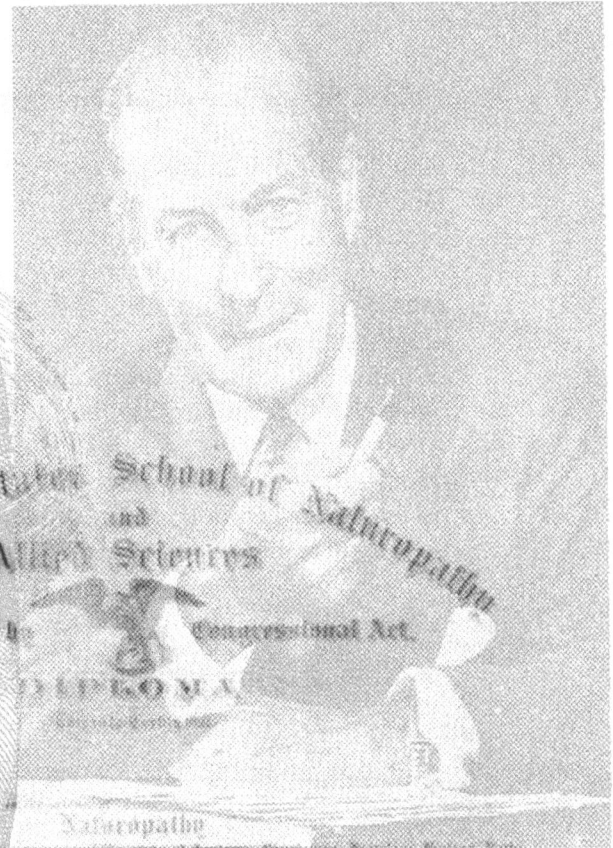

The United States School of Naturopathy
and
Allied Sciences

DIPLOMA

DOCTOR OF NATUROPATHY

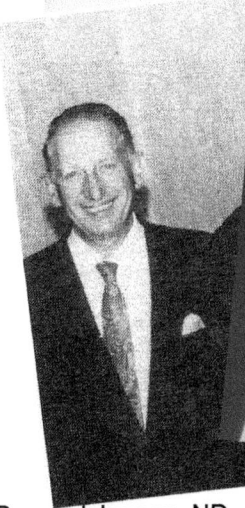

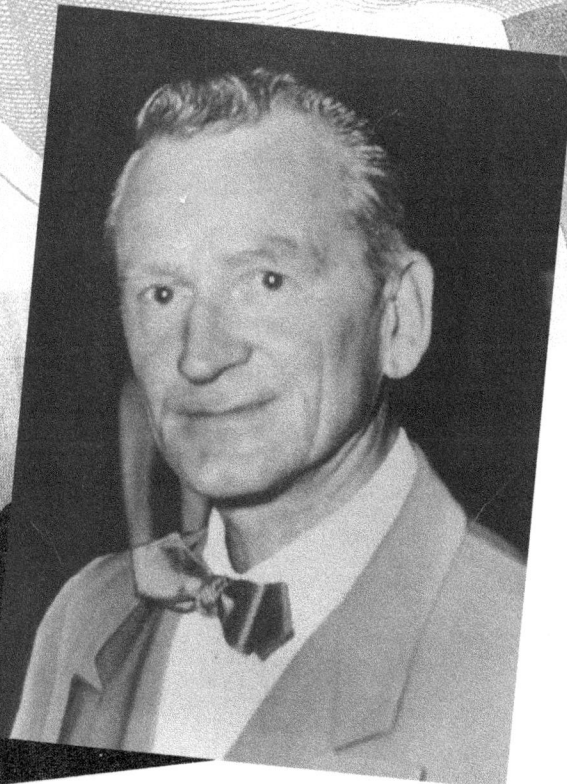

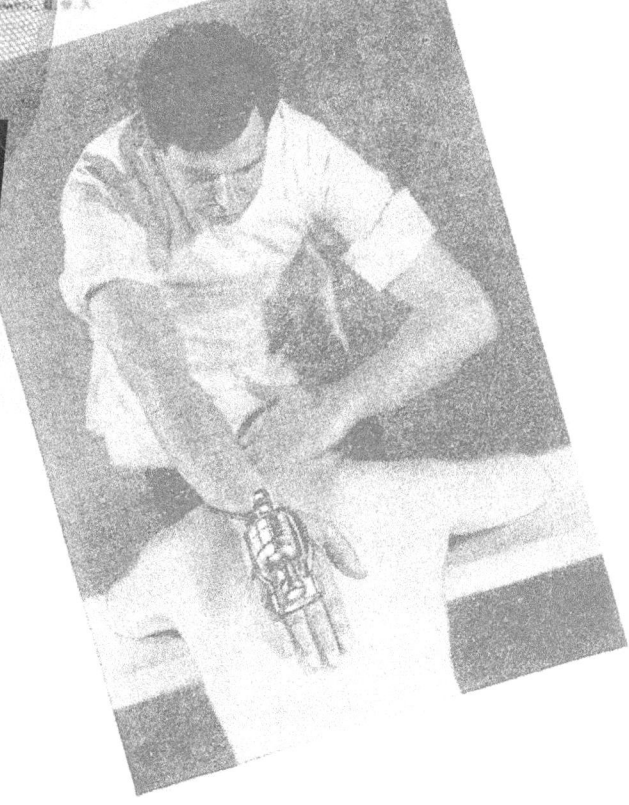

Bernard Jensen, ND   William Turska, ND (AP wirephoto 1960)

1960–

- **United States School of Naturopathy,** the last surviving college of Frederick Collins' First National University, begins offering the **Doctor of Naturopathic Medicine (NMD)** degree in addition to its ND degree that it has offered since 1910. Relocated to Washington, D.C., and under the direction of Dr. Hyman Goldberg and Dr. Civet Kristal, the school institutes an expanded curriculum and more rigorous examinations for the NMD degree. Nevertheless, the curriculum adheres to a strict traditional naturopathic model and not a pseudo-medical model, despite the inclusion of the word "medicine" in its degree.

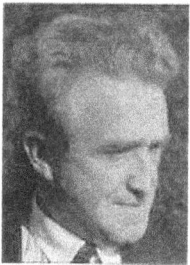

- **James C. Thomson, ND dies.** He was one of the founders of the Society of British Naturopaths and the Incorporated Society of Registered Naturopaths. He was considered "the Scottish Lindlahr".

- **National College of Naturopathic Medicine moves to Seattle,** Washington. It retains an "extension division" in Portland, however.

1961–

- **Frank B. Hamilton, ND,** takes over editorial duties on *American Naturopath*, the monthly journal that for decades would be politically independent and called for unity among all organizations and types of naturopaths.

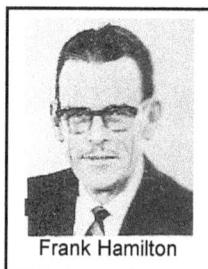

Frank Hamilton

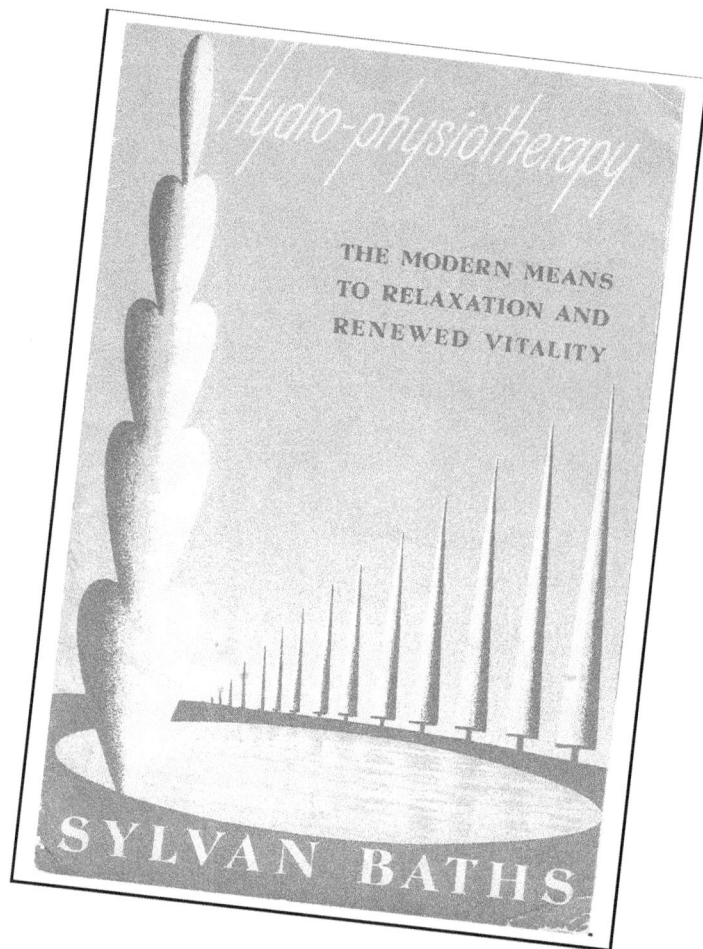

Hydro-physiotherapy

THE MODERN MEANS TO RELAXATION AND RENEWED VITALITY

SYLVAN BATHS

By this time, the methods that were originated by the naturopaths, such as hydrotherapy, were passing into more wide use as elective therapies in the spa environment. Institutions such as Sylvan Baths in New York City offered many therapies that, formerly, the presiding ND would have prescribed. On the other hand, places like the Libbey Physical Medicine Clinic in Hot Springs, Arkansas maintained a clearly medical purpose.

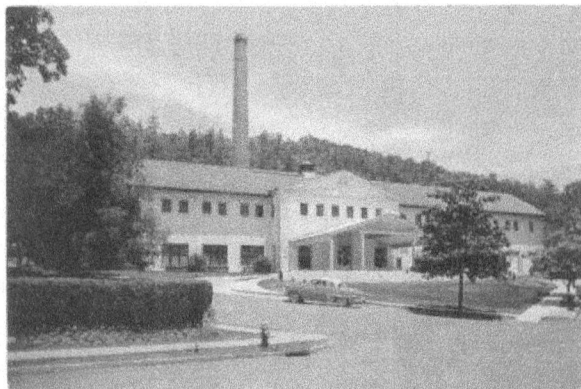

Equipment for hydrotherapy in the Fordyce Bath
House (Hot Springs, Arizona) along with gymnasium.

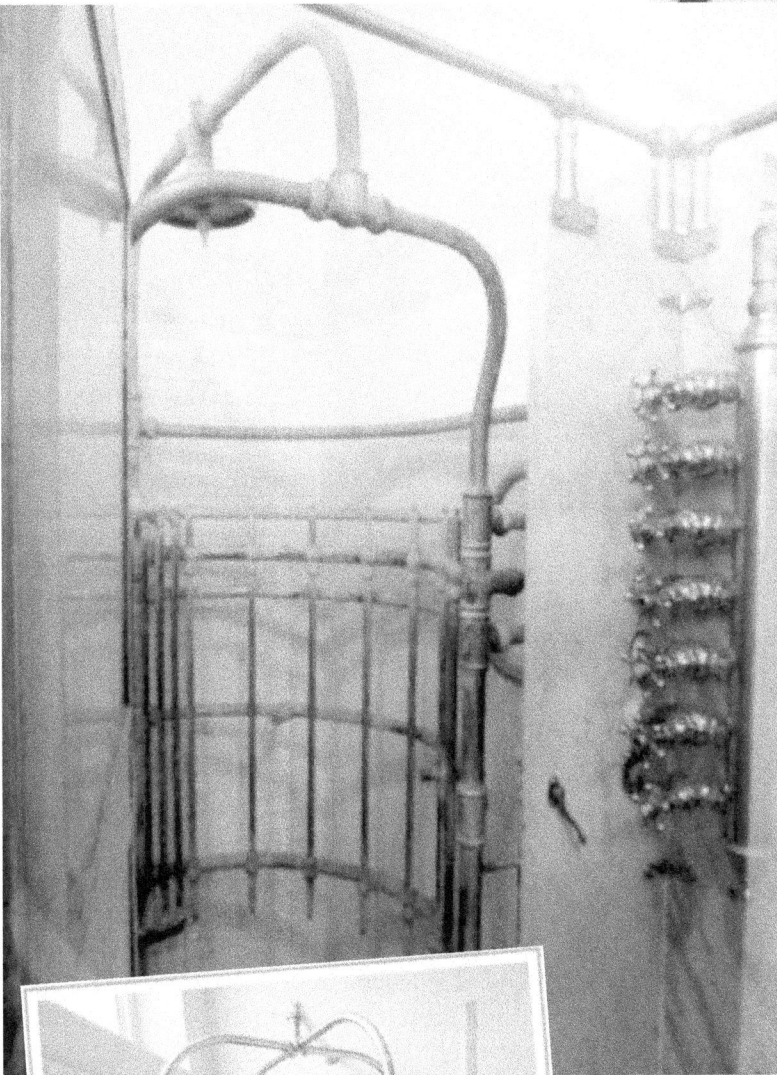

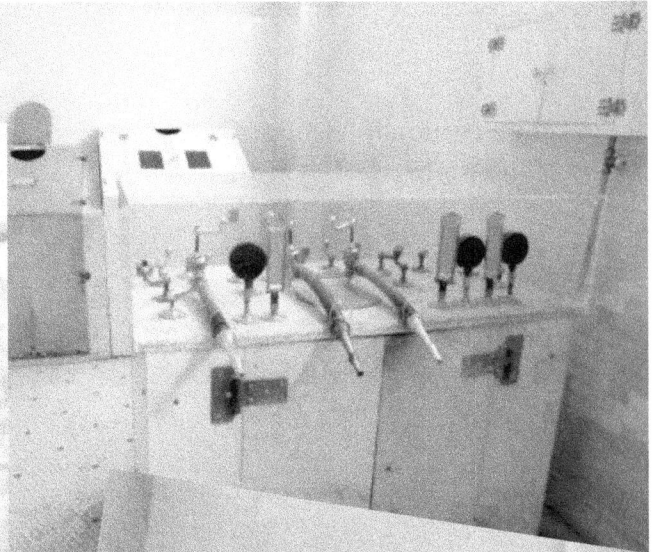

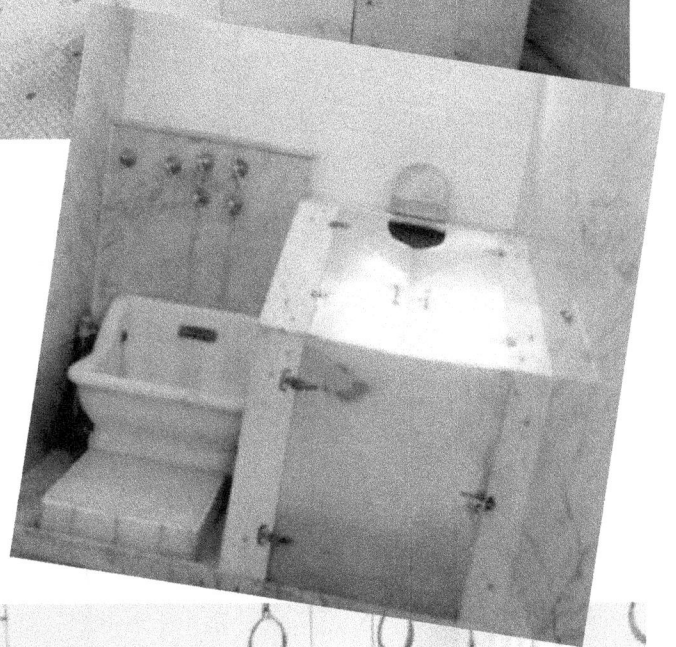

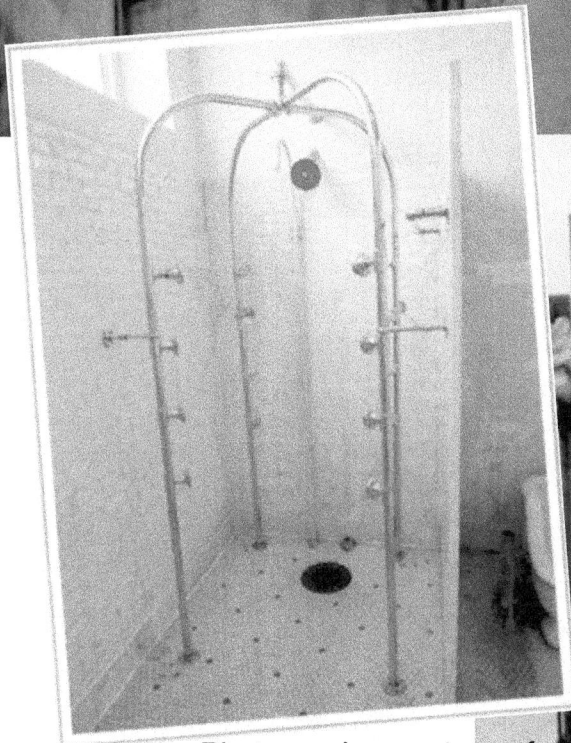

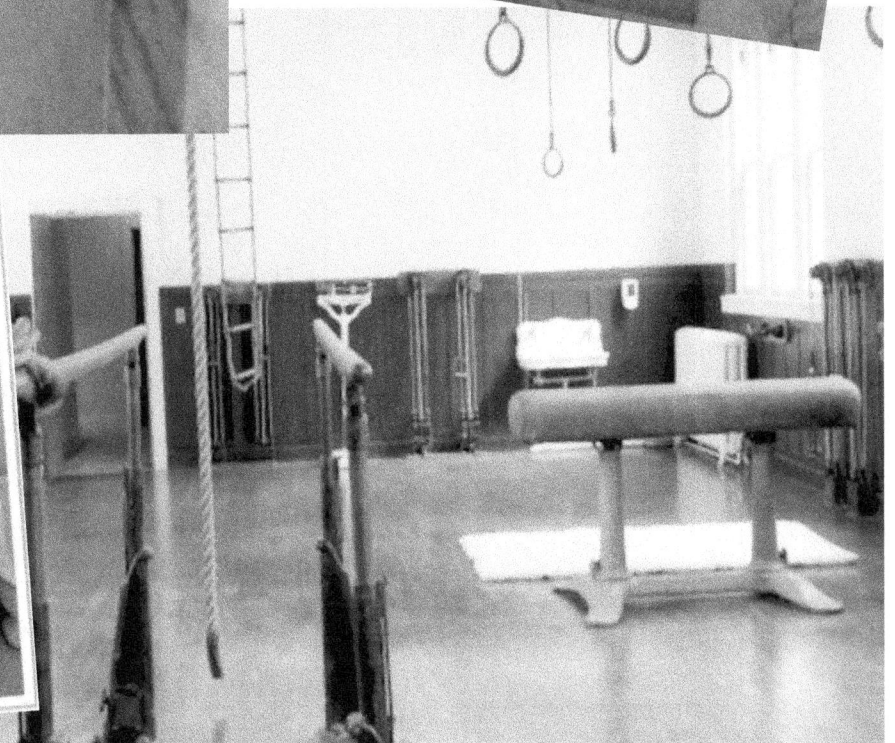

Photographs courtesy of
George Yuhasz, ND

- **The National Association of Naturopathic Physicians (NANP)** begins publishing their journal, calling it *The Naturopath*. Although this is virtually the same title of Benedict Lust's longtime publication spanning decades, no acknowledgment is made of this legacy. Editor John Noble declares its December 1962 premiere to be the first appearance of the title.

A 1910 issue of Benedict Lust's *The Naturopath*

The NANP claims *The Naturopath* is a new publication

- **Stanley Lief, ND dies** at age 72 due to residuals from a childhood heart defect. The most famous of the naturopathic pioneers in England, he was sent there to take over an institution (previously run by Bernarr MacFadden) after studying Naturopathy in the United States. Lief was born in Russia but spent most of his life in the U.K.. He established the original and largest English nature cure establishment *Champney's* (which would be used as a background setting in the James Bond film *Thunderball*). Leif, in addition to his many other accomplishments developed his own variation on the practice known in Naturopathy as "Bloodless Surgery", and called it "Neuromuscular Therapy". It is still a popular modality in massage therapy. He was elected president of the Nature Cure Association of Great Britain and Ireland in 1932 and was active in various organizations after, including the British Naturopathic Association. He established the College of Naturopathy in 1949. Leif was known as "the British Lust" for his organizing work in establishing Naturopathy in England.

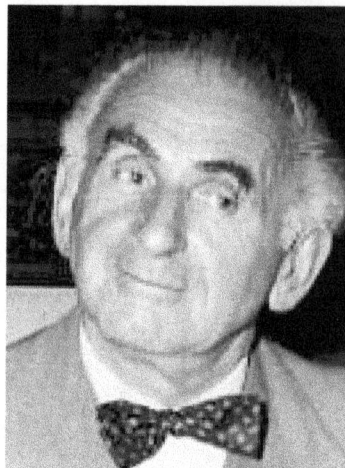

- **Otis G. Carroll, ND dies.**

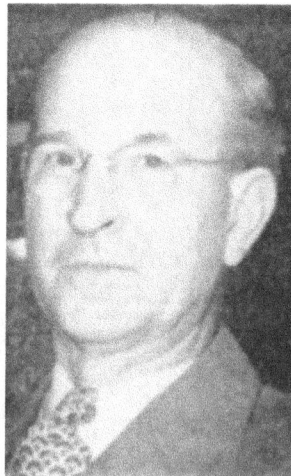

He was one of the most outstanding naturopaths of the Twentieth Century and had practiced in Spokane, Washington since 1917. His methodology centered on hydrotherapy, dietary regulation, botanical medicines, and homeopathic medicines.

Cured of arthritis at an early age by Dr. Alex LeDoux (a practitioner trained by Father Kneipp himself), he was inspired to become a naturopath and studied with Dr. LeDoux, and later attended Lindlahr's College of Naturopathy in Chicago. He returned after graduation to Washington and set about revising the typical way of applying contrast hydrotherapy. Over the years, he developed what he called "Constitutional Hydrotherapy", which created a powerful systemic response, and reduced the length of time necessary to apply it. With his final version, a treatment could be applied in the office in only 45 minutes or so. Carroll had a number of trained attendants to apply the treatments to a countless number of patients who filed in and out of his clinic every day.

He was a very skillful botanical prescriber and amazed other naturopaths who came to study with him by the number of plant medicines he knew thoroughly. But in application, he used very simple compounds of two or three herbs for short periods, such as his "42 Cocktail" (four parts Artemesia, two parts Aloe) to clear the intestinal tract. He kept his patients supplied with some of these simple combinations, instructing them in their use. He was also a skilled homeopath.

His other unique contribution to Naturopathy was his Carroll Food Intolerance Test, in which he was able to determine the foods, and combination of foods, that were acting as triggers for the patient's illness. Poorly digested and assimilated foods, Carroll realized, were the obstacles to complete cure by other naturopathic methods. He modified the Abrams electronic method to detect these intolerances, and he began curing his most difficult cases--the first being his son, who had not responded to anything. Dr. Carroll said, "Health must at all times come from, and be maintained by, digested foods."

He was the brother of Robert Carroll, ND, one of the architects of the pseudo-medical direction that naturopaths in the Pacific Northwest first began pursuing in the late 1940s. The two brothers had a strained relationship due to the difference in their philosophies and methods.

His methods would be carried on by his son Bill, and by Leo Scott, ND, and Harold Dick, ND, who both apprenticed under him..

1964–

- **California "sunsets" its naturopathic licensing law.** While previously licensed NDs may still practice, no new licenses will be issued. Conventional medicine's opposition to Naturopathy has been more visible in recent years by the vigorous lobbying to rescind laws licensing NDs.

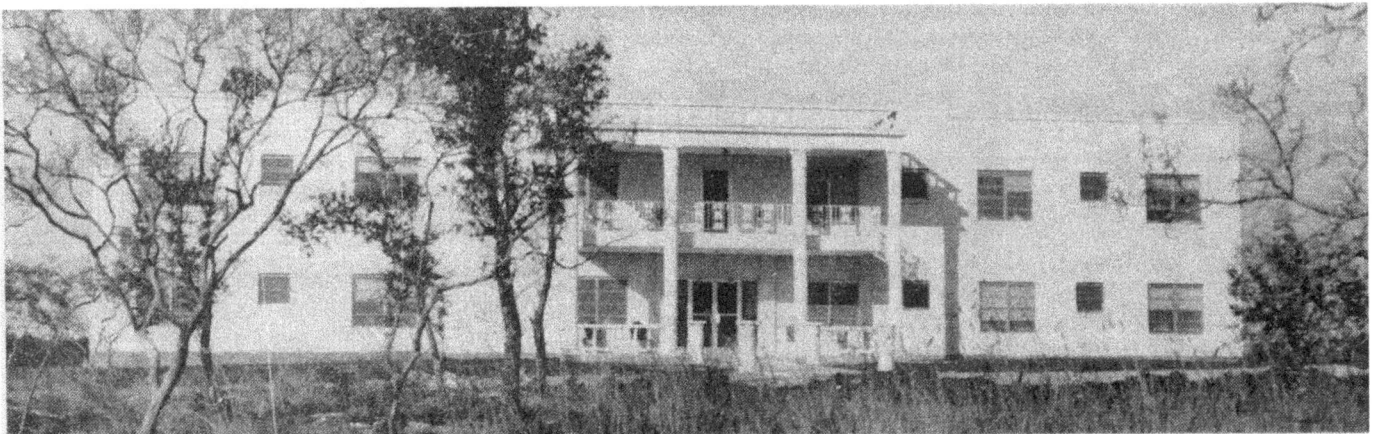

Dr. Shelton's Health School, San Antonio, Texas. Herbert Shelton ND, who broke with the naturopathic mainstream years before, has operated a fasting and detoxification facility for 45 years and conducted thousands of therapeutic fasts. He publishes the monthly *Hygienic Review*, teaching healthy living. The magazine's slogan is "Let Us Have The Truth, Though The Heavens Fall."

PROFESSIONAL DIRECTORY OF NATUROPATHIC PHYSICIANS

BRITISH COLUMBIA
CLOVERDALE

ROBERT FLEMING
B.Sc., B.T.Sc., N.D.
18375 Trans-Canada Highway
R.R. 3 — Tel. 574-4811
Cloverdale   B.C.

MONTANA

DR. MARCEL R. PITET,
B.A., N.D.
Naturopathic Physician
General Practice
259-5774   702 Broadwater
Billings, Montana

NEW YORK

DR. J. W. NOBLE, N.D.
Naturopathic Physician
1920 N. Kilpatrick St.
BU 9-6544

DR CHARLES R. STONE
Internal Botanical Medicine
X-Ray Diagnosis, Minor Surgery

SALEM

DR. R. REYNOLDS CLINIC
Rectal Disorders
Phone 363-9460
1144 Center Street   Salem

DR. JOSEPH A. ROMBOUGH
General Practice
JU 1-2364
1305 Summer St. N.E.   Salem

Fasting
Weight-reducing
Natural Hygiene
Boating / Swimming
Sports
Library

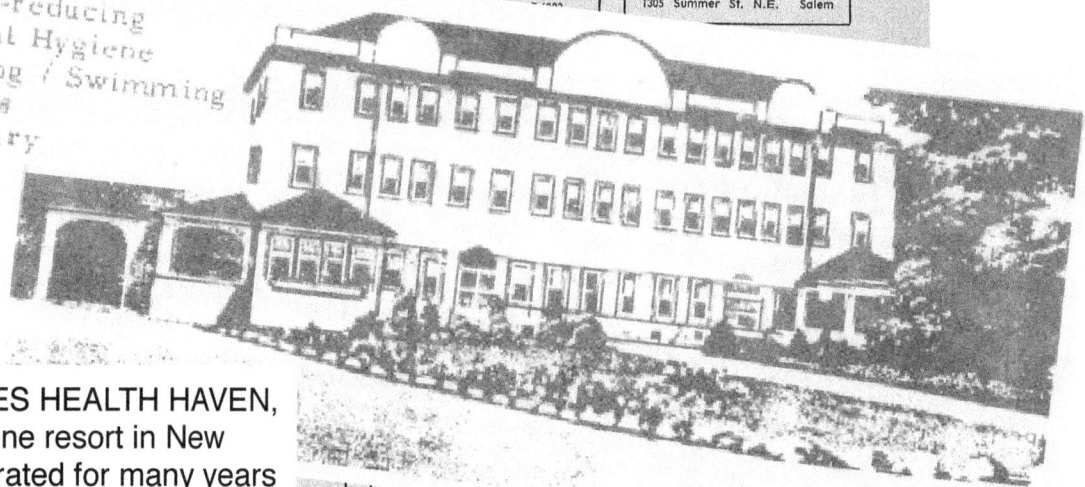

LIFE SCIENCES HEALTH HAVEN,
a natural hygiene resort in New
York state operated for many years
by Stanley Bass, DC, ND

General Practice
926 N.W. Tualatin Valley Hwy.
MI 4-4000

Phone 343-9302
108 N. Latah   Boise

...atment
Facilities - X-Rays - Laboratory
Electrotherapy - Diets - Herb
Formulas - Electrocardiography
3619 S.E. Division   BE 5-0333

DR. HENRY R. LINKE, N.D.
Naturopathic Medicine, X-Ray
and Manipulations
Kellogg, Idaho

DR. FRANKLIN HEISLEY
Colon and Stomach Disorders
Rectal Diseases - Arthritis and
Rheumatism - X-Ray - Physio-
therapy - Colonic Irrigation
Complete Clinic Facilities
4160 S.E. Division   BE 6-2927

MEDFORD

RALPH R. WEISS, N.D.
Diagnosis, Clinical Nutrition, Botanical Medicine, Posture Correction, Physiotherapy
Phone 772-9713
426 Medical Cent. Bldg., Medford

Adjustments, Cabinet
Colonic Irrigations, Arthritis,
Rheumatism, Digestive Disorders
E. A. MATZ, N.D.
cor. Main & Tower   736-4154
Centralia, Washington

FALL CITY

JERRY G. MARTINEZ, N.D.
Castle 2-4909
Fall City   Wash.

INDIANA

DR. R. RICHARD STAUB
Naturopath
Bio-Chemical Therapist
108 W. 12th St.   Ph. 267-7735
Winona Lake, Indiana

DR. GEORGE C. JOHNSTON
Naturopathic Physician
315 N. E. 94th Ave.   AL 4-1198

REDMOND

DR. MAURICE M. PENDROY
7th and Black Butte
Phone 548-2531   Redmond

SEATTLE

CYRUS E. MAXFIELD, N.D.
Naturopathic Physician
Hours: Mon., Wed., Fri., 9 to 5:30
Thursday by appointment
Phone CH 3-5252
Seahurst Naturopathic Center
1835 S.W. 152nd St., Seattle 98166

The NATUROPATH
408 POSTAL BUILDING
PORTLAND 4,

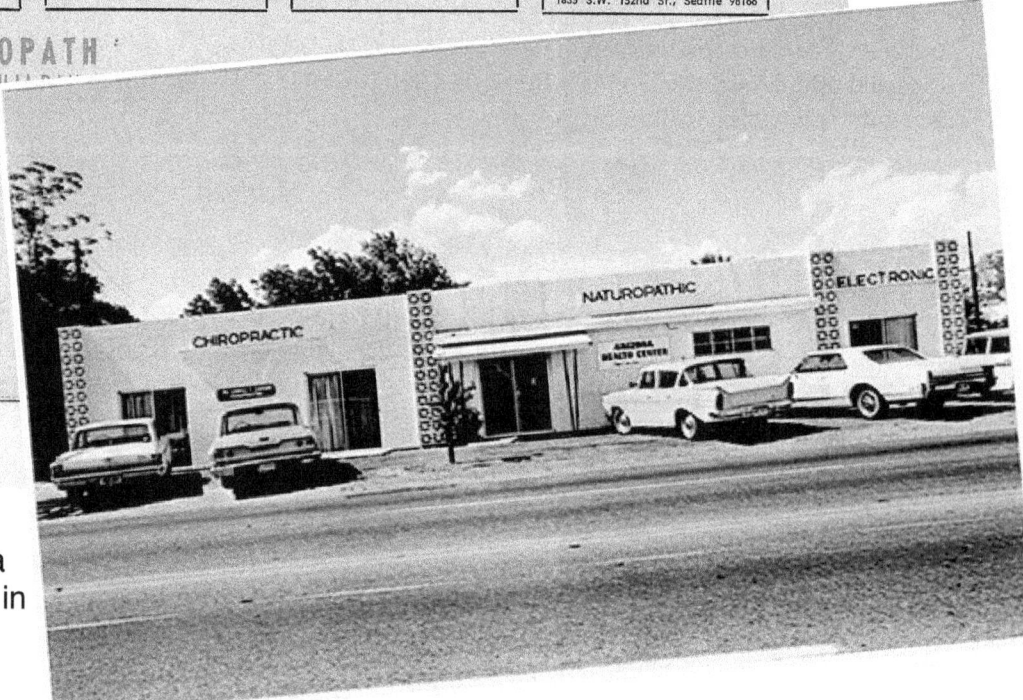

An Arizona clinic offering a
range of natural therapies in
the early '60s.

1965–

- **Only eight states in the U.S. now license naturopaths, out of twenty-three during Naturopathy's golden age.**

- The British Naturopathic Association becomes the **British Naturopathic and Osteopathic Association**. The British College of Naturopathy and Osteopathy in North London granted both the ND and the DO degrees at the end of its four-year program (The Osteopathic Association of Great Britain, however, would not accept the ND/DO licensees in their register).

1967–

- **Max Otto Garten, DC, ND** writes *Health Secrets of a Naturopathic Doctor*, which puts the subject of naturopathic methods back in the public eye.

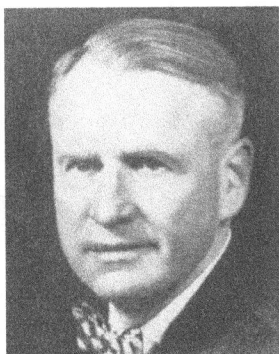

1968–

- **The training of new naturopaths continues to decline.** National College of Naturopathic Medicine enrolls only seven students for this academic year (three will go on to graduate).

Meanwhile, natural medicine is still going strong in Europe. The British College of Naturopathy and

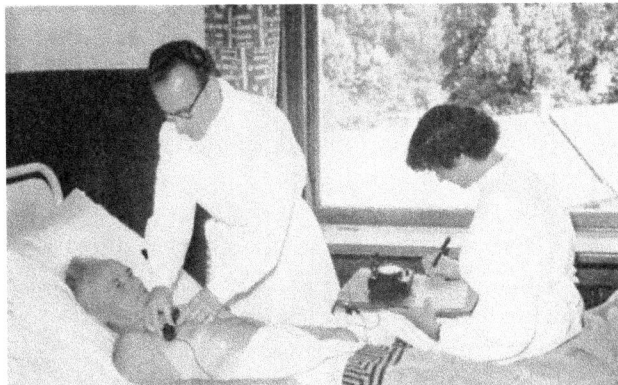

Osteopathy has an abundance of graduates, as seen below.

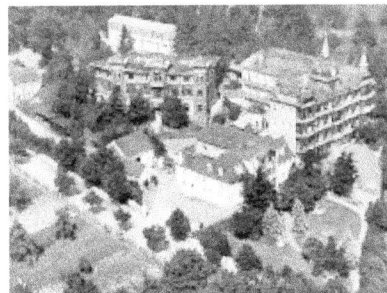

Patients staying at institutions like this clinic at **Worishoven, Germany**, have competent medical monitoring but are treated with natural therapeutics. There is a much greater respect for naturopathic methods in Germany, the birthplace of the movement.

The Bilz Sanatorium, founded by Freidrich Bilz (detailed in Chapter One) still stands in its magnificence. The Dresden facility continues to draw people to its healing therapies in the 1960s, more than a half century after its establishment.

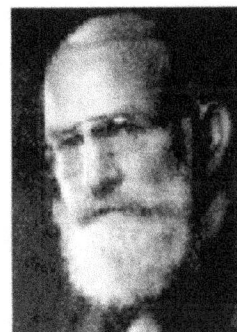

Germany was not the only place famous for natural cures. **Maximilian Bircher-Benner, MD**, operated a sanatorium in Zurich, where he used nature cure methods and was considered the "John Harvey Kellogg of Switzerland". He was also the inventor of *muesli* cereal. Bircher-Benner's clinic became famous for its cures of chronic diseases all over Europe, and would be in existence until the 1990s. **Henry Lindlahr** studied there with Bircher-benner in the early 1900s.

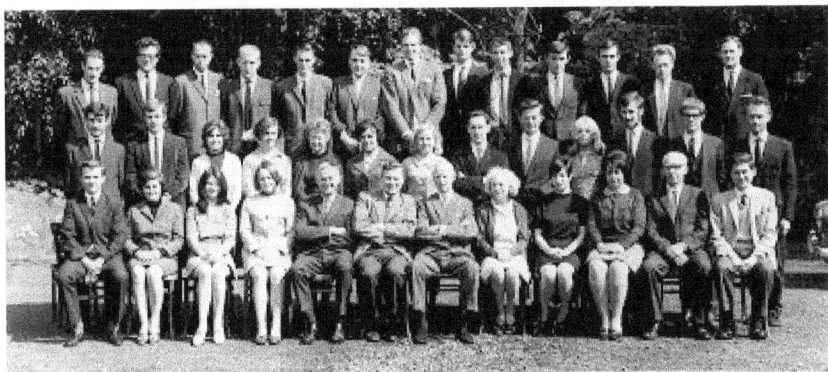

1968–

- **Paavo Airola, PhD, ND, writes** *There IS a Cure for Arthritis*, based on naturopathic research in Europe and elsewhere.

Airola, born in Finland, studied naturopathy in England and Sweden. A graduate of the British College of Naturopathy and Osteopathy, he was a member of the British Guild of Drugless Practitioners. He studied biochemistry and nutrition and attended numerous natural medicine clinics in Germany, Sweden, and Switzerland, including Bircher-Benner's. He lived for a time in Canada, where he began compiling data for his books.

Dr. Airola moved to America and settled in Phoenix, Arizona. Because of the paucity of knowledge regarding nutrition and low-tech natural methods within conventional medicine, he became a popular visiting lecturer at many medical schools, including Stanford University Medical School. His continuing education seminars were well regarded despite the fact that he was a naturopath.

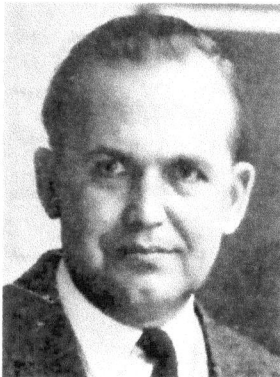

He gave many Americans their first picture of what was being done in naturopathic clinics and sanatoriums in Europe at a time when such institutions had disappeared in the U.S.

Airola popularized the term "biological medicine" to describe such methods. He would go on to write a number of best-selling popular books on natural medicine.

1969–

- **M.O. Garten, DC, ND** writes *The Natural and Drugless Way to Better Health*.

- **Gerald E. Poesnecker, DC, ND becomes director of the Clymer Clinic** in Pennsylvania, which becomes one of the best-

known facilities providing natural medicine in the country. R. Swiburne Clymer, MD dispensed rational medical advice and used natural therapeutics, and became regionally renowned for it before bringing in Poesnecker as director. A graduate of National College of Naturopathic Medicine, Poesnecker appears and the clinic takes on a distinctly naturopathic flavor. He will ultimately preside over a team of forty-five various healthcare providers. Many other clinics would model themselves after the Clymer Clinic in the years to come.

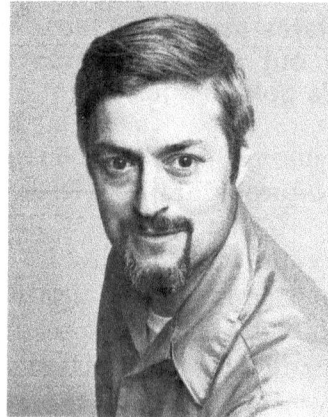

Gerald Poesnecker, ND

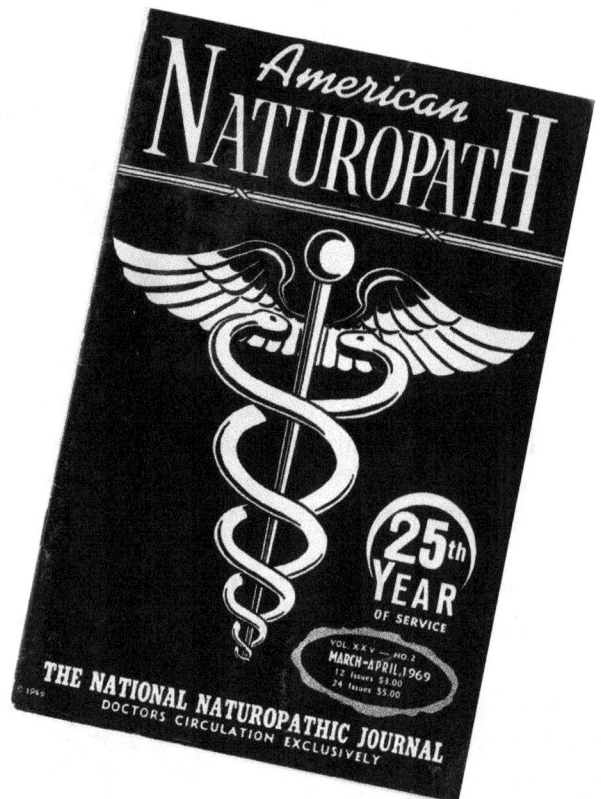

American Naturopath is still in print in 1969.

- The Indian government agency, the Ministry of Health and Family Welfare, establishes the **Central Council for Research** in Ayurveda, Yoga, Naturopathy, Unani, Siddha, and Homeopathy in 1969.

1970—

- **Prof. Hilton Hotema, DC, ND** dies at the age of 92. Hotema was at one point a partner of Herbert Shelton, and involved in the development of the Natural Hygiene movement, a subset of Naturopathy. Hotema wrote many books on longevity, most of them veering into the mystical. His original, purely naturopathic, work was *The Law of Life and Human Health* (1926), which he wrote under his birth name, George Clements.

1971—

- *Are You Confused?*, **a new book by Paavo Airola, ND** appears. It sorts out valid and questionable health practices for an eager public without access to naturopathic doctors. The market for self-empowering health books is growing rapidly, and Airola is one of its best-selling authors.

1973—

- **Washington State limits scope of practice of naturopaths** to dietary advice and massage.

1974—

- *How To Get Well,* a primer for laypeople using naturopathic principles to better their health, is authored by Paavo Airola, N.D. It becomes a perennial bestseller. Airola ultimately wrote fourteen popular books on natural medicine and health.

- **Harry Hoxsey, naturopath and heir to the herbal cancer formulas handed down in his family, dies** in Texas. Hoxsey once operated cancer clinics in seventeen states before the FDA had them all closed. Despite this, the National Cancer Institute concluded after tests that the Hoxsey formulas did in fact cure several types of cancer. Hoxsey was the only naturopath to successfully sue the American Medical Association and its director for its persecution and slander against natural medicine. His last remaining clinic, in Baja California, would remain in operation into the next century, despite regulations that prevent shipping the Hoxsey medicines to the U.S.

1975—

- **National College of Naturopathic Medicine** enrolls 63 students, up from only 23 the year before. A resurgence begins in the natural medicine profession.

- **G.E. Poesnecker, DC, ND writes** *It's Only Natural,* a book for patients that explains all the different naturopathic modalities in use at his clinic. It provides a snapshot of the eclectic methods in use by Poesnecker's generation of naturopaths, before conventional medical methods begin filtering into the naturopathic educational process.

- **The Australian Naturopathic Practitioners Association** is formed.

1976—

- **John W. Noble, ND dies.** He was one of the principal founders of National College of Naturopathic Medicine, and first editor of *The Naturopath*, a journal in print from 1963 to 1980.

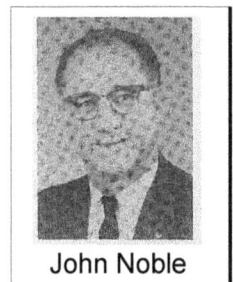

John Noble

- **The Seattle location of National College of Naturopathic Medicine closes.** A dearth of students and financial woes made it necessary. The school had moved to Washington state in 1959.

1977—

- **National College of Naturopathic Medicine relocates again,** back to Portland, Oregon.*

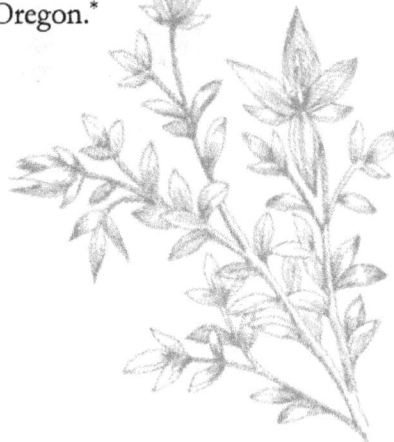

1977—

- **Jesse Mercer Gehman, ND, once president of the American Nautropathic Association, dies.** A lifelong physical culturist, his early bodybuilding led him to be the model for the statue of Columbus at the Columbus Monument in his hometown of Reading, PA.

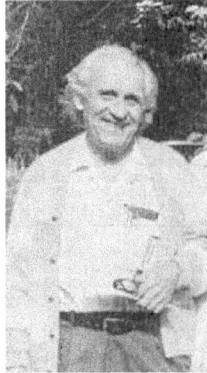

Following the death of Benedict Lust, Gehman was appointed President of the Eastern ("parent body") ANA. Some time later, there would be a struggle for control between Gehman and Paul Wendel, ND, who insisted that *he* had ascended to the presidency, and for a while there would be two factions of the Eastern ANA, leading to Gehman's use of the appellation "parent body" to describe the organization with an unbroken tie to the original Lust association. Following the death of Gehman, Theresa M. Schippell, ND would assume the presidency of the Eastern ANA.

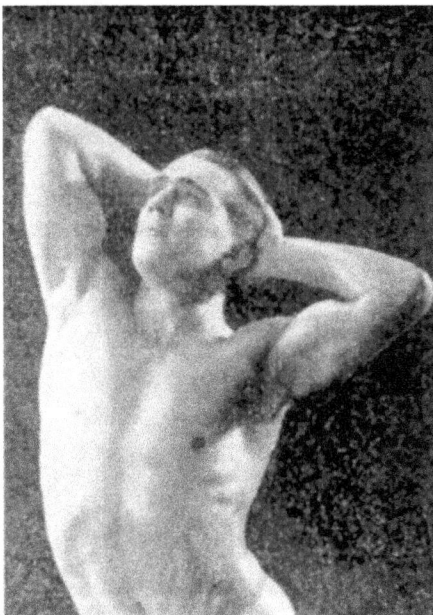

A young Jesse Mercer Gehman

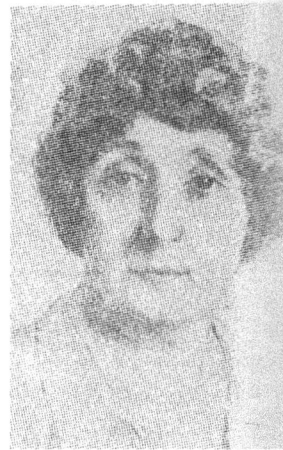

T.M. Schippell, ND

Schippell almost single-handedly brought about naturopathic licensure in the District of Columbia, due to her treating the Hon. Katherine Langley, who then introduced and fought for a naturopathic licensing bill.

She was a trusted and valued aide to Benedict Lust and was on the board of directors of the ANA for many years. She would write a regular column in *The Naturopath and Herald of Health* for years after the death of Lust, in the space Dr. Lust's column formerly occupied. Another example of Naturopathy's tradition of sexual equality, Dr. Schippell was committed to the original course of Naturopathy and the ANA as set down by the founder, but found it more and more difficult to maintain membership in the original organization in the face of the dynamic public relations of the "other" ANA, controlled by the Western group. By the time the pseudo-medical community went through its evolution from Western ANA to "American Naturopathic Physicians and Surgeons Association" to "American Association of Naturopathic Physicians" to "National Association of Naturopathic Physicians" (in 1955), Dr. Schippell had worked for organization and expansion among the traditional naturopathic ranks. Now, with the death of Gehman, the task would rest solely on her shoulders.

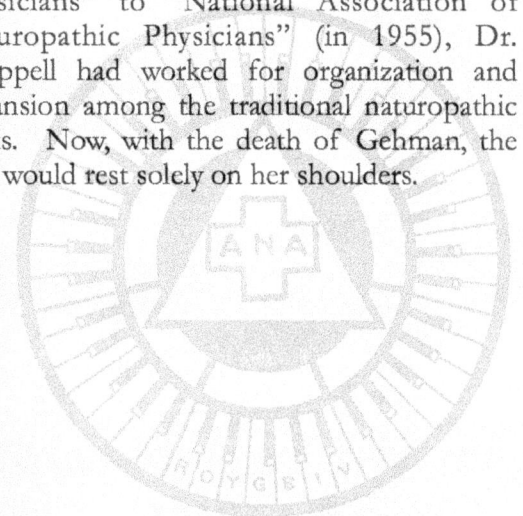

6

THE MODERN DIRECTION

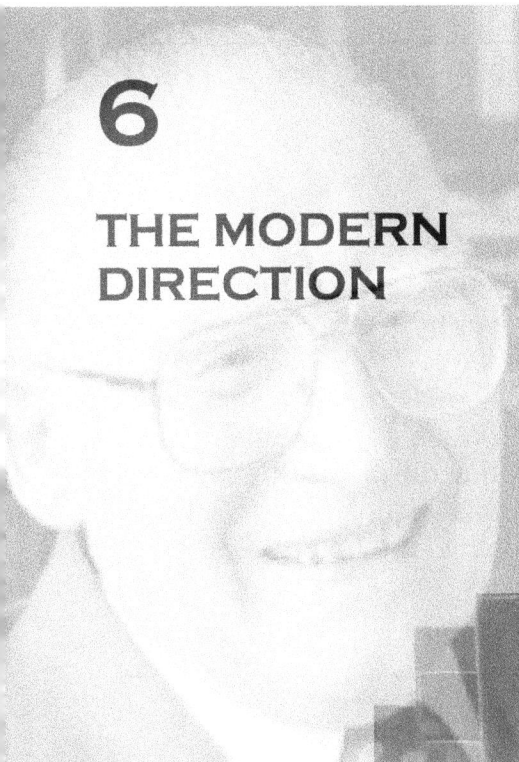

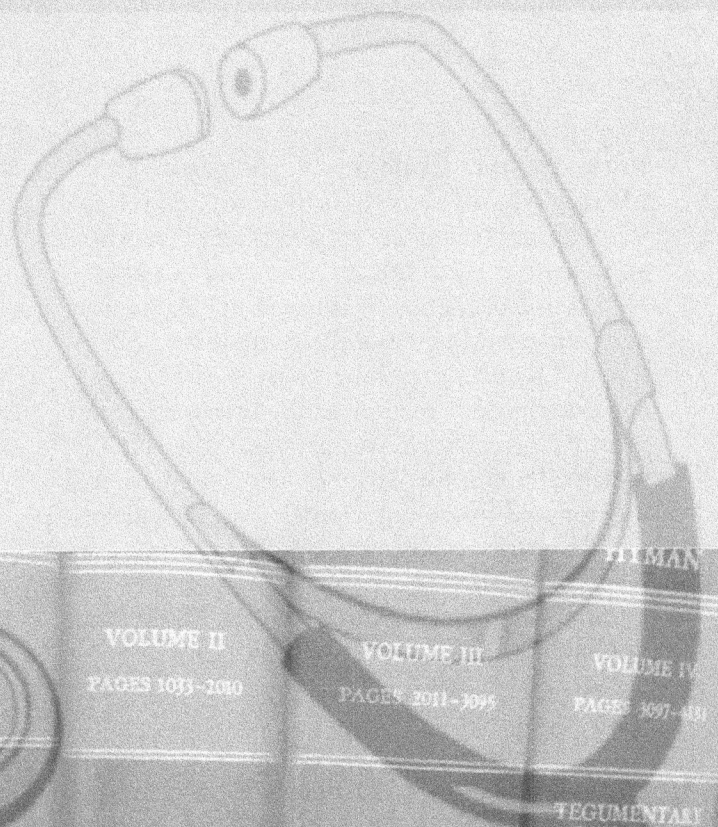

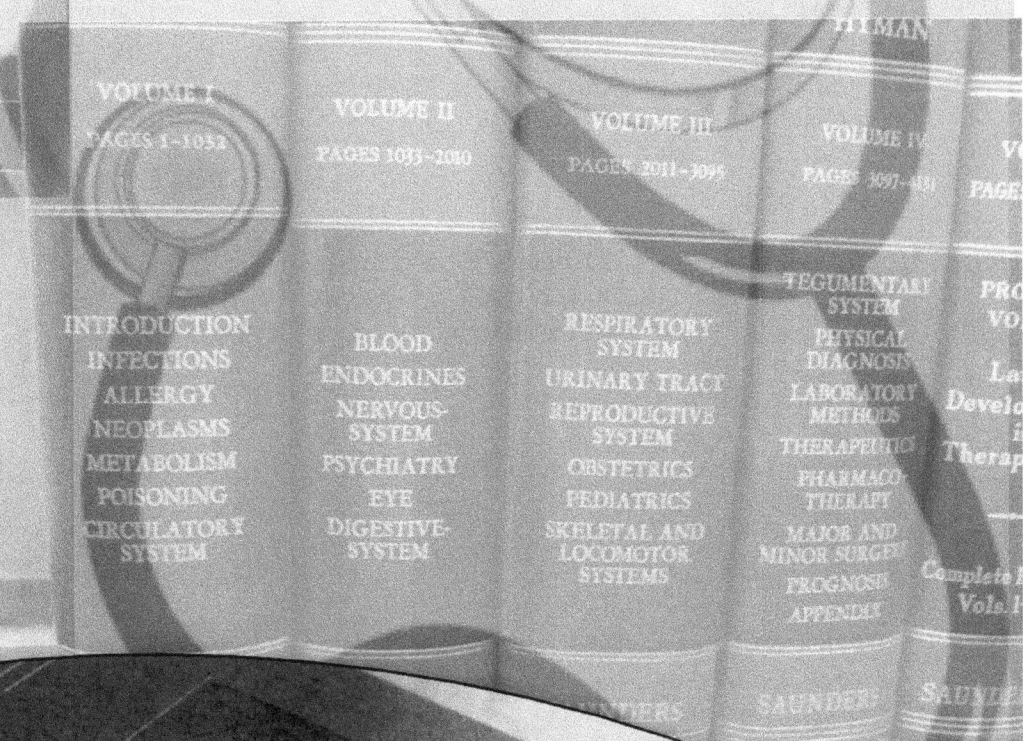

VOLUME I
PAGES 1–1032

VOLUME II
PAGES 1033–2010

VOLUME III
PAGES 2011–3095

VOLUME IV
PAGES 3097–...

VOLUME
PAGES

INTRODUCTION
INFECTIONS
ALLERGY
NEOPLASMS
METABOLISM
POISONING
CIRCULATORY
SYSTEM

BLOOD
ENDOCRINES
NERVOUS-
SYSTEM
PSYCHIATRY
EYE
DIGESTIVE-
SYSTEM

RESPIRATORY
SYSTEM
URINARY TRACT
REPRODUCTIVE
SYSTEM
OBSTETRICS
PEDIATRICS
SKELETAL AND
LOCOMOTOR
SYSTEMS

TEGUMENTARY
SYSTEM
PHYSICAL
DIAGNOSIS
LABORATORY
METHODS
THERAPEUTICS
PHARMACO
THERAPY
MAJOR AND
MINOR SURGERY
PROGNOSIS
APPENDIX

Complete
Vols.

SAUNDERS

SAUND

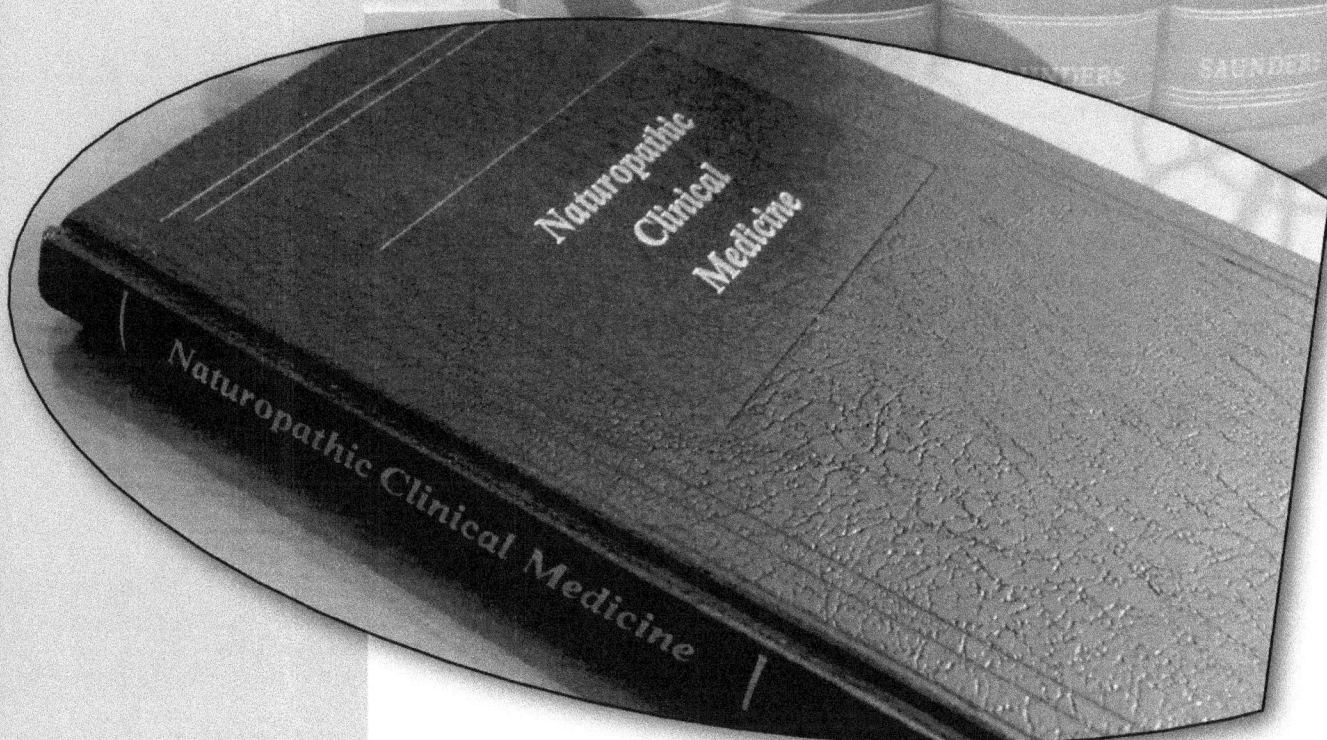

Naturopathic
Clinical
Medicine

Naturopathic Clinical Medicine

1978—

- **John Bastyr College of Naturopathic Medicine is established** in Seattle, Washington. Founders are Joseph E. Pizzorno and Lester Griffith, 1975 graduates of National College of Naturopathic Medicine, and William Mitchell, a 1976 graduate. The fourth organizing member was Sheila Quinn, an experienced medical administrator from nearby University of Washington. The school is named for John Bartholomew Bastyr, their mentor and instructor from National College of Naturopathic Medicine.

- **Pacific College of Naturopathic Medicine opens** in Monte Rio, California. Faculty is derived mostly from DC/ND graduates of the old Western States College.

- **Ontario College of Naturopathic Medicine opens** in Kitchener, Ontario, Canada. Initially it would be a postgraduate institution for MDs, DCs, and NDs from other programs who wished to add to their credentials.

- **The National Association of Naturopathic Physicians** offers "three-day intensive courses on homeopathic medicine". ♦

- **Four class action suits** designed to restore or initiate licensure in Idaho, Texas, North Carolina, Maryland, Michigan, Wyoming, and Alaska is brought by the National Association of Naturopathic Physicians and several state associations. It was initiated by officials of the NANP, including Joseph Pizzorno, John Bastyr, William Sensenig, William Turska, David Shefrin; and also medical doctors like psychiatrist Clifford Passen, MD (who was granted an ND), and Timothy Dooley, an ND who also became a medical doctor.

The suits alleged that an illegal monopoly had been created by orthodox medicine and that naturopaths' constitutional rights had been violated. Named as defendants were various state medical and pharmacy examining boards, the U.S Department of Health, Education, and Welfare, and the Food and Drug Administration. The suits were lost, appealed, and lost again with a Supreme Court decision.* 98

Meanwhile, elsewhere…

Government Nature Cure Hospital, a 60-bed facility, is established in Kirala, India. Traditional naturopathic methods are used without an allopathic staff or facilities.

In 1978, the Ministry of Health and Family Welfare separates the various natural medicine councils under its jurisdiction, with Naturopathy and Yoga in one distinct department and Homeopathy in another.

1979—

- **Arizona College of Naturopathic Medicine, a branch of the American University of Natural Therapeutics, closes** in Bisbee, Arizona.

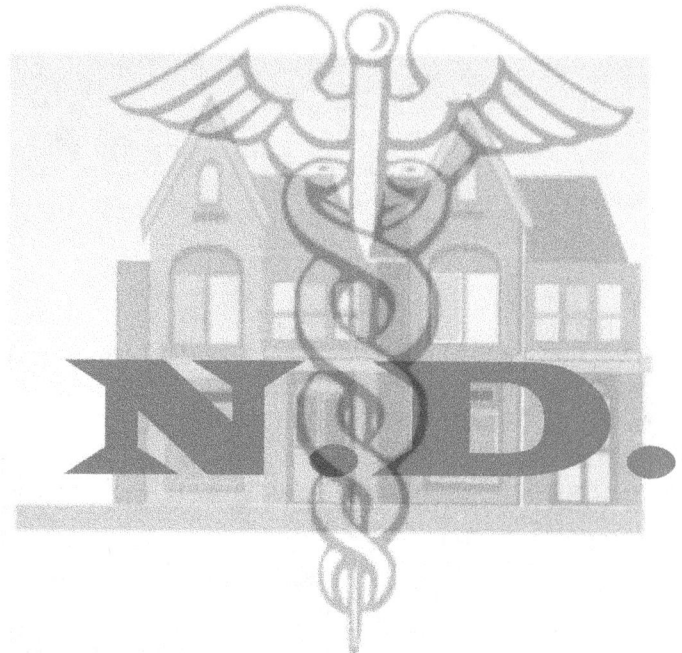

♦ *Digest of Chiropractic Economics*, July/Aug 1978, p. 101

* Nos. 77-1346, 77-1908, 77-2593, 77-2594, United States Court Of Appeals, Fourth Circuit, 582 F.2d 849; 1978 U.S. App. LEXIS 9326

1980—

A survey reveals only 175 licensed naturopathic doctors still practicing in the U.S. Licensing laws have been repealed or "sunsetted" in all but three states by this time. Although many unlicensed naturopaths are still in practice (many are "grandfathered") in many states, those in the Northwest are the most scrutinized for census purposes, and form the majority of the 175 counted. They will form the vanguard for the rebirth of the licensed ND. The others will be ignored in the years to come, to reinforce the historical view that naturopathic doctors were at one time almost extinct. The truth, as would be unraveled years later, is that NDs who were not practicing in a pseudo-medical manner were simply struck from the rolls. Surveys such as these do not reveal an accurate picture of those days, but served an agenda that gave an impetus to the establishment of new schools that, in addition to creating a resurgence of natural medicine, would create an entirely new "green allopathic" version of the profession.

- **The seminal school that would become Clayton College of Natural Health opens** in Birmingham, Alabama. Founded by Dr. Lloyd Clayton, DC, ND, it is a distance-learning school that will become the best known of its kind. Its Doctor of Naturopathy program will graduate the largest number of naturopaths of any institution over the years to come. The proliferation of Clayton graduates will cause the school to be vilified by the emerging pseudo-medical naturopaths as personified by National and Bastyr graduates.

- **Once again, a name change: The National Association of Naturopathic Physicians (NANP) dissolves in financial ruin.** After bankruptcy, the principals of the organization plan to re-group. Jim Sensenig, academic dean at National College of Naturopathic Medicine, Kenneth Blanker, President of the Nevada Naturopathic Medical Association, and Mel

Shelton, president of the Federation of Naturopathic Licensing Boards, organized a meeting in Nevada to create a new organization called the **American Naturopathic Medical Association**. Bernard Steuber was elected President, Richard Thurmer, Vice-President, and Donald Hayhurst, Secretary/Treasurer.

It is speculated at the time that the change in name, rather than injecting new life into the old organization, is adopted in order to distance the principals from the taint of controversy surrounding the former attempts by the NANP in 1978 to force legislators to restore naturopathic licensure in many states where they had been repealed. They were not successful in this. Insiders said this was partly due to a number of scandals involving the alleged selling of diplomas by the two schools overseen by the organization. Many legislators and lobbyists were reputedly disenchanted with the group, and a new name and new faces would make for better public relations in the second round of trying to re-establish the profession.

1981—

- **A second "American Naturopathic Medical Association" (ANMA) organization is founded**, this time uniting traditional naturopaths and those with other degrees who practice natural medicine. It represents the traditional counterpart to the pseudo-medical ANMA. It is founded by Donald Hayhurst, ND.

Hayhurst was a naturopathic activist in Nevada when the first ANMA was formed; he attended the first organizational meetings and was elected Secretary-Treasurer. He differed in viewpoint from the others partly because he was trained prior to the founding of the pseudo-medical schools. He did not support medically based education for naturopathic students. The others also took issue with his endorsement of modalities that the new bio-medically oriented naturopaths wanted to exclude from standard practice, such as iridology. Hayhurst adopted the same organizational name and rallied the increasingly disenfranchised traditional naturopaths to join together.

He would go on to lead the largest naturopathic organization in the country, the second ANMA.* Noting that the first organization with that name never filed its incorporation papers or bylaws, Hayhurst incorporated his group while the first ANMA was essentially non-functioning.

> "We need standards and we need more—to stand by them, once they are established…these standards should insist on a thorough training in basic nature Cure. All students should be required to be thoroughly competent in applying the methods of the old masters…Our standards should include thorough training through the study of Kneipp, Preissnitz, Just, Kuhne, Rikli, Trall, Schroth, Graham, Jennings, Lust, and MacFadden…We need adequate standards for entrance upon training for a Doctorate in Naturopathy, but these standards need NOT be, nor should they be patterned after, the medical requirements."
>
> --Jesse Mercer Gehman, ND; speech to the eastern ANA, 1947❖

These words, although spoken more than 30 years earlier, could not have described better the viewpoint of the new traditional naturopathic organization, the ANMA.

1981—

- **Pacific College of Naturopathic Medicine closes its doors** before graduating its first class. The California school was financially challenged from the start. Credits are accepted by Bastyr and National until July 1982. Students are faced with the necessity of relocating to either Washington or Oregon.

- **National College of Naturopathic Medicine purchases a new school facility,** along with seven acres of land, in Portland.

* American Naturopathic Medical Association web site

❖ Quoted in Freibott, *Pseudomedicalism: Naturopathy's Demise?*, (report submitted to the U.S. Department of Education)

1982—

- **National College of Naturopathic Medicine opens its new outpatient clinic** on the school premises.

1983—

- **Dr. Paavo Airola dies** at age 64 of a cerebral hemorrhage in Finland, a result of complications from injuries sustained during his emigration after World War II. He authored fourteen books on natural medicine and health, and popularized the term "biological medicine".

- **Ontario College of Naturopathic Medicine expands its program** to a full four-year curriculum, based on that of National College in Oregon and Bastyr College in Washington. The biomedical orientation of the new program causes a split in the naturopathic community, much like the U.S., where those with a "nature cure" approach complained about the inclusion of allopathic material. British Columbia naturopaths protested that such an orientation was discriminatory because it required conventional medical education as a prerequisite for naturopathic schooling.

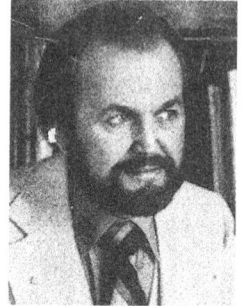

- **John R. Christopher, ND dies** from head trauma after slipping on ice at the age of 73. Christopher studied at Dominion Herbal College in Vancouver, BC and became a Master Herbalist in 1946. In 1948 he received his ND from the Institute for Drugless Therapy in Iowa. Concentrating on botanical medicines, he developed a reputation for curing incurable cases. He practiced for many years in Utah, where he was harassed by the medical establishment and hauled into court five times, winning in each case. The state eventually passed a law prohibiting him from practicing. Dr. Christo-

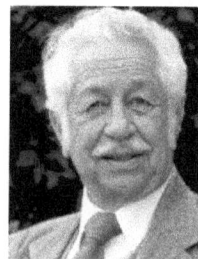

100

pher was more responsible than any other one person for the survival of herbal practice during the decline of the naturopathic profession. His teaching of botanical medicines to the lay public, however, set him apart from other NDs, and the new generation did not recognize him as the senior expert he was. But he was a consultant to the retail herbal industry in its early years, and his botanical formulas have been available in health food stores for decades. Christopher founded the School of Natural Healing in Springville, Utah in 1953.

- **The World Health Organization (WHO) recommends the integration of naturopathic medicine** into conventional health care systems.

1984—

- **Ontario College of Naturopathic Medicine moves** to Toronto.

1985—

- Name changes again!
  The first American Naturopathic Medical Association, representing the pseudo-medical NDs, finding itself in stark competition with the other ANMA, changes its name back to an earlier appellation, American Association of Naturopathic Physicians (AANP). The original AANP was a short-lived body that never achieved any prominence. The new AANP would continue to represent the new generation of progressive, pseudo-medical naturopaths, with no confusion as to identity. James Sensenig is President, and Kathy Rogers is Vice-President.

  An organization by this name had been formed and incorporated in Indiana in 1941 and was intended to be a national society, but did not reach any eminence. Now, however, the principals of this group sought to establish themselves as not only the progressive national organization, but the *only* national organization. No references to the original American Naturopathic Association or the International Society of Naturopathic Physicians—both still in existence—would be made from then on in

the AANP's transactions. Their considered enemy would be the American Naturopathic Medical Association (ANMA), led by Don Hayhurst.

- **Norman Walker, ND, dies** at the age of 99. He was the most widely known exponent of raw foods and juicing. He advocated drinking fresh raw fruit and vegetable juices, and invented the Norwalk hydraulic juice press, which is still one of the highest quality juicers available. At one time Walker ran a health ranch in Arizona, and he wrote a number of popular health and nutrition books, including *The Natural Way To Vibrant Health*, *Become Younger*, and *Colon Health: The Key To A Vibrant Life*. Walker was still physically and mentally fit when he died peacefully during a nap.

1986—

- **Westbrook University commences its distance-learning courses**, including its naturopathic program. It will go on to train 7,000 NDs by the second decade of the Twenty-first Century.

"Naturopathy does not make use of synthetic or inorganic vitamins or minerals, or of drugs, narcotics, surgery, serums, vaccines, anti-toxins, toxoids, injections or inoculations."

(Re-affirming the definition of Naturopathy at the Golden Jubilee convention in 1947, by the American Naturopathic Association

---

DESPOTISM

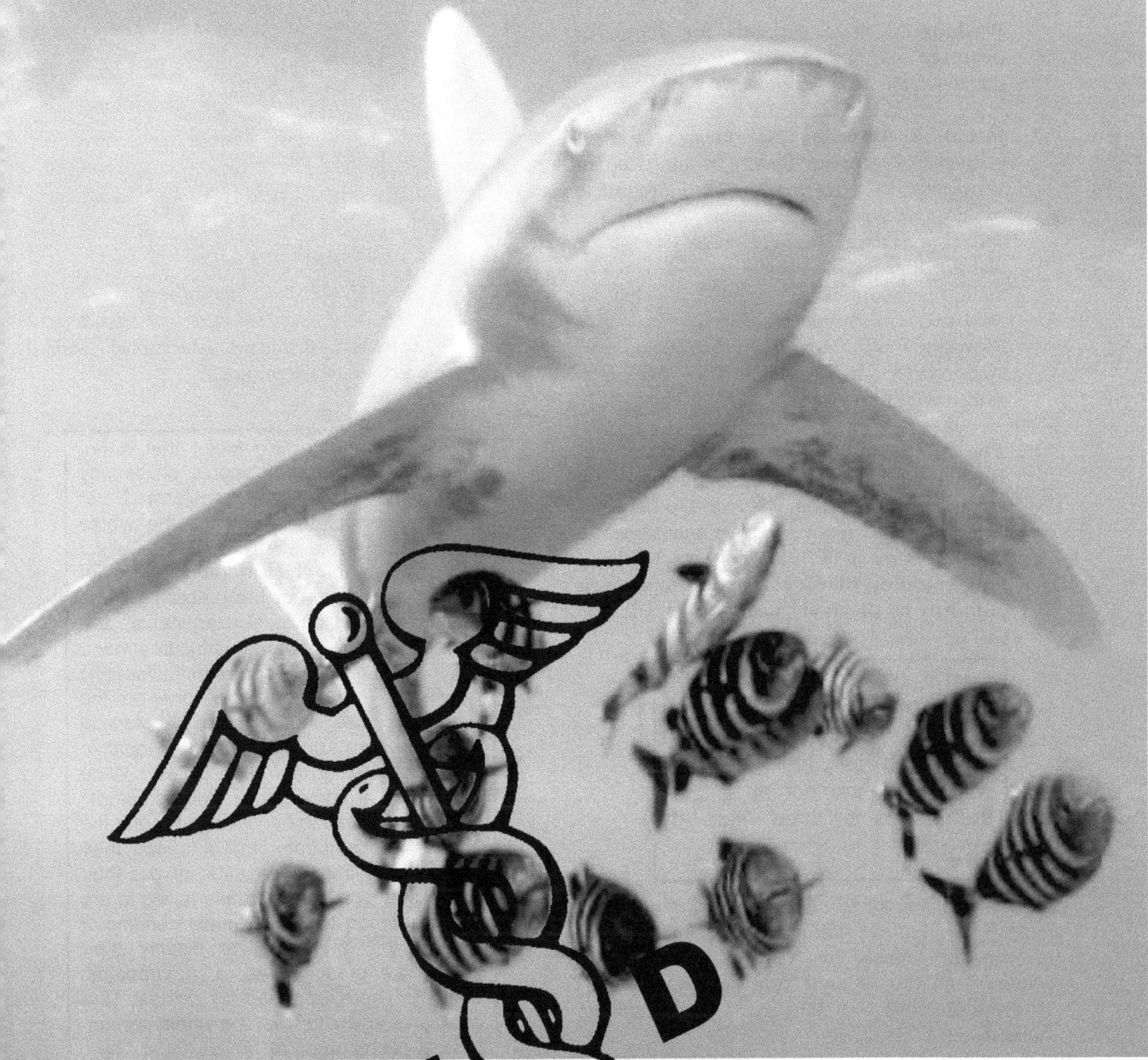

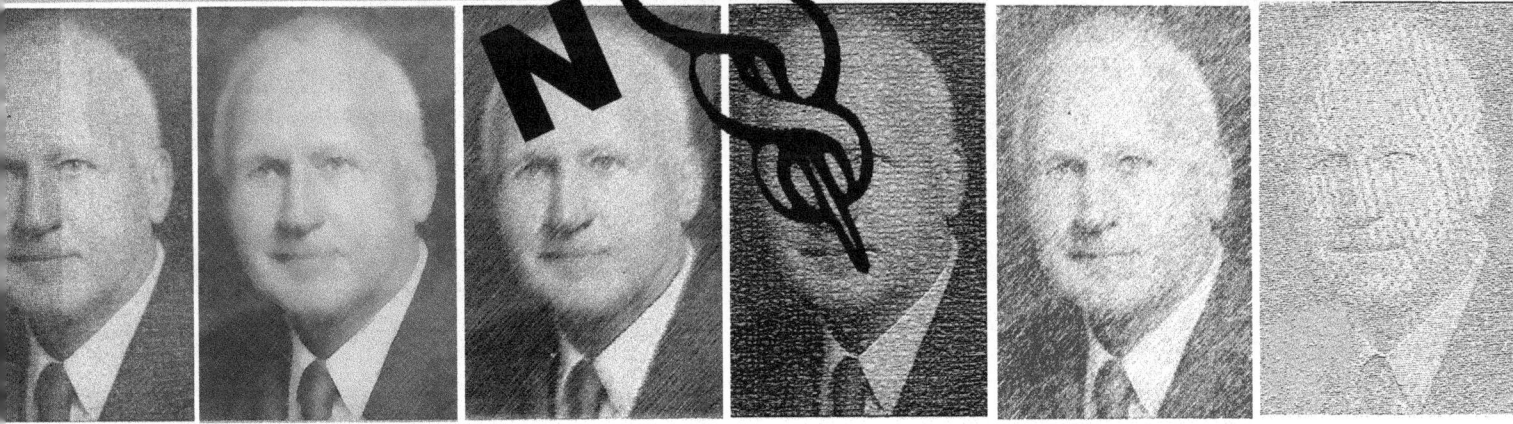

1987—

- **Washington State expands the scope of practice** of naturopaths to all natural therapies, and allows diagnostics.

- **Joseph A. Boucher, ND dies.** A 1954 graduate of Western States, he practiced in Vancouver, BC. He was one of the founders of the Canadian Naturopathic Association, and also a founder of National College of Naturopathic Medicine, where he taught for many years. Influenced mainly by Tilden, he used the Schroth system of detoxification as his major tool. Today's Boucher Institute of Naturopathic Medicine in British Columbia is named after him.

- **The Council for Naturopathic Medical Education (CNME) is organized** by graduates of Bastyr and National colleges; it applies for and receives recognition from the U.S. Department of Education. **Schools of long standing object to the assumption of authority by this body,** which credentials only two schools—National and Bastyr.

> Bastyr College, the flagship institution for the new naturopathic direction, was developed by three doctors who had been out of school themselves for three years at most.

The curricula at the CNME-accredited schools will now follow a model similar to that of medical and osteopathic schools: two years of basic science courses and two or more years of clinical work. Prerequisite college of three years is required for admission.*

Also, graduates are required to take the two-part NPLEX national board examination after the second and fourth years. This establishes them as candidates for licensure by those states that do license naturopathic doctors. Those naturopaths who took other national board exams, however, are increasingly not eligible for licensure, nor will they be allowed to sit for the NPLEX.

* *Council on Naturopathic Medical Education Accreditation Handbook*, 2007 edition

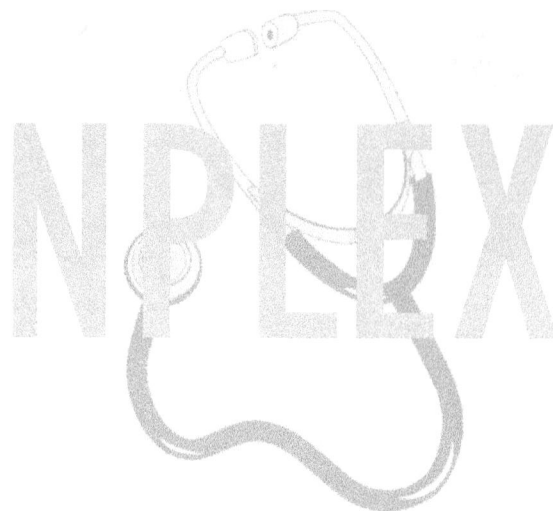

Years later, a criticism of this new educational standard will be the only one to see print:

> "NPLEX is another big factor that is not aligned with our profession's philosophy and either must be transformed, or removed completely. Firstly, the whole examination system of NPLEX is an exact reproduction of the allopathic way of medicine. Except for the practical exams testing skills in physical examination and in each modality of naturopathic treatment, the NPLEX is filled with allopathic questions. Even the questions on the modalities like nutrition and botanical medicine are posed in an allopathic manner. How do you treat colitis? What is a good treatment plan for migraines, ADD, constipation? Nowhere on the NPLEX are students tested to see their rapport with their copatients, to put their good listening skills and case-taking to the test, to demonstrate their understanding of naturopathic principles, to display their creative expression as a naturopathic doctor. There is especially no test of a clinician's ability to treat the whole person, to treat each person as an individual..."
>
> --Daniel Block, ND
> *The Revolution of Naturopathic Medicine*, 2003 Collective Co-op Publishing, Page 96

MINIMIZATION vs. MEDICALIZATION

Polarization progresses as the two major naturopathic camps each move farther from the median: Modernists, calling themselves *naturopathic physicians*, adopt an unabashedly conventional medical training, including biomedical sciences, synthetic drugs, and surgery. Naturopathic methodology is still taught in the colleges, but mostly in introductory courses with fewer hours than schools earlier in naturopathic history.

Their opponents, calling themselves *traditional naturopaths*, return to a more basic Nature Cure format, discontinuing many therapies that naturopaths used to perform and instead acting as health and lifestyle coaches. Gone are the hydrotherapies, joint manipulation, light therapy, and electric stimulation used by an earlier generation of NDs. Dietary counseling, recommendation of vitamins and exercise, and instruction in self-application of various therapies by the client take their place.

Lost in the picture of this conflict is a third group. Graduates of schools now closed or on their last legs, trained in a wide array of natural medical techniques, were what are referred today to as *classical* **or** *original* *naturopaths*. Most of them well trained in medical subjects but rejecting an allopathic or conventional

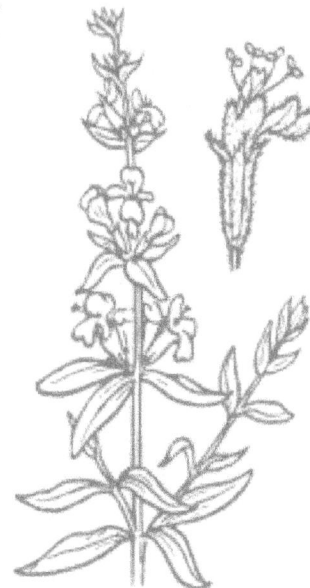

approach to treatment, some had previous medical training at non-naturopathic schools and used bridge programs to complete their schooling to receive their naturopathic diplomas. These NDs were to have no descendants. The schools maintaining the original standards of training had mostly fallen by the wayside by this time. A few limped along. United States School of Naturopathy and Allied Sciences (founded by Collins) and Central States College (founded by Spitler), two of the Class A schools of the 1940s, were among the very few to still exist with a curriculum that trained naturopaths who were considered *physicians* and not health counselors, but who did not seek to copy any practices of the medical doctor.

Classical naturopaths have been written out of history by extremists on both sides.

Pseudo-medical naturopathic schools tell their students that they are the equivalent of medical doctors, and all other NDs are inadequately-trained graduates of diploma mills. Traditional naturopaths often make the claim that they are practicing true Naturopathy by simply educating people about health, and denounce the use of the terms *medicine* and *physician* in conjunction with it.

Neither group makes reference to the many schools that turned out competent general practitioners who functioned as doctors—but stopped short of using allopathic medical methods.

Following is a list of naturopathic colleges, most of which existed before the field was dominated by the CNME schools. Most have closed or are inactive. Some reach back to the profession's infancy and others are of more recent origin. They are arranged alphabetically.

1. Academy of Natural Healing (Santa Fe, NM)
2. American College of Naturopathic Medicine (Salem OR)
3. American School of Naturopathy (New York, NY)
4. American School of Oriental and Homeopathic Therapy (Miami Beach, FL)
   (Note: the school name changed to Pan American School of Natural Medicine)
5. American College of Natural Medicine (Salem, OR)
6. American College of Naturopathic Medicine and Laboratory Technic (Kansas City MO)
7. American Therapy University (Arcadia, MO)
8. American University of Natural Therapeutics (AZ)
9. Anglo-American Institute of Drugless Therapy (London, England)
10. Arizona College of Naturopathic Medicine (Bisbee, AZ)
11. Bernardino College of Natural Medicine (Claremont, CA)
12. California College of Natural Healing Arts (Los Angeles)
    (Note – this school was absorbed by Los Angeles College of Chiropractic, Glendale, CA)
13. California College of Natural Medicine (Ventura, CA)
14. Central States College of Physiatrics (Eaton, OH)
15. Clayton College of Natural Health (Birmingham, AL)
16. Clayton University (St. Louis, MO)
17. College of Drugless Healing and Naturopathy (Los Angeles, CA)
18. College of Drugless Physicians/National College of Chiropractic/Naturopathy (Chicago)
    (Note: this school was renamed the National University of Health Sciences; recently (2006) it began offering training in Pseudo-Medicalist Naturopathy; Lombard, IL)
19. College of Naturopathic Physicians and Surgeons (Los Angeles, CA)
20. Columbia College of Chiropractic Naturopathic program (NYC)
    (Note: this school merged with New York Chiropractic College in the mid-1950s)
21. Eastern College of Neuropathy and Naturopathy (Philadelphia, PA)
22. Emerson University (Los Angeles, CA)
    (Note: this school was formerly called the California University of Liberal Physicians)
23. Florida College of Integrative Medicine, Naturopathic Program (Orlando, FL)
24. Florida College of Naturopathic Medicine (Bradenton, FL)
25. Gateways College of Naturopathy and Natural Therapeutics (Shingle Springs, CA)
26. Gem State College of Naturopathic Medicine & Surgery (Twin Falls, ID)
27. Golden State University (Los Angeles, CA)
28. Hallmark Naturopathic College (Sulphur, OK)
29. Hollywood College of Naturopathic Physicians and Surgeons (Hollywood, CA)
30. I.W. Lane College (Winter Park, FL)
    (Note: this school today teaches allied health courses)
31. International College of Naturopathy (name changed to California College of Natural Medicine) (Ventura, CA)
32. John Thomas College of Naturopathic Medicine (St. Charles, MO)
33. Lincoln College of Naturopathy (Indianapolis, IN)
34. Metropolitan College of Chiropractic, Naturopathic Program (Cleveland, OH)
35. Minneapolis College of Naturopathy (MN)
36. Missionary College of Naturopathic Medicine (City/State not confirmed)
37. Missouri Institute of Naturopathy (St. Louis, MO)
38. Nashville College of Naturopathic Medicine (Nashville, TN)
39. National College of Chiropractic/Naturopathy (Chicago)
    (Note: see also #15: College of Drugless Physicians/National College of Naturopathy)
40. National School of Naturopathy (Cedar Rapids, MI)
41. Natural Therapeutics College (Mesa, AZ)
42. National University of Therapeutics (Washington, DC)
43. New Mexico School of Natural Therapeutics (Santa Fe, NM)
44. New York College of Naturopathy (NYC)
45. North American College of Natural Health Sciences (Mill Valley, CA)
46. Northwest Drugless Institute (WA)
47. Philadelphia College of Naturopathy (Philadelphia, PA)
48. Pacific College of Natural Medicine (CA)
49. Santa Fe College of Natural Healing (Santa Fe, NM)
50. Sierra State University College of Naturopathic Medicine (San Francisco, CA)
51. Southern California College of Chiropractic and College of Naturopathy
52. Southern College of Naturopathic Medicine (Brownsville TX)
53. Southern University of Naturopathy and Physiomedicine (Miami, FL)
54. St. Louis College of Physicians and Surgeons (St. Louis, MO)
55. Texas College of Naturopathy (Dallas, TX)
56. United States School of Naturopathy and Allied Sciences (Newark, NJ and later Fort Oglethorpe, GA)
57. Universal Sanipractic College (WA)
58. University of Natural Healing Arts, College of Naturopathy (Denver CO)
59. University of Natural Medicine (San Dimas, CA)
60. Westbrook University (distance learning)
61. Western College of Chiropractic and Drugless Therapy (San Francisco, CA)
62. Western States Chiropractic College, Naturopathic Program (Portland, OR)

Pseudo-medical Schools:
1. Bastyr University (Kenmore, WA)
2. National College of Natural Medicine (Portland, OR)
3. National University of Health Sciences (Lombard, IL)
4. Southwest College of Naturopathic Medicine (Tempe, AZ)
5. University of Bridgeport (Bridgeport, CN)

When one reads the revisionist history put forth by both the CNME-accredited schools and also the traditional naturopathic community, many of these schools and their long list of graduates are strangely missing. To hear the one camp tell it, licensing laws were repealed, *all* schools finally closed, and the profession was almost extinct until rescued by a few visionaries who resurrected it and raised its standards.

The story told in the other camp is that those same pseudo-medical "visionaries" initiated a lobbying campaign to restore licensure in states that had rescinded it, pursued litigation against the states when they did not comply, and incurred the displeasure of the Attorney General in each state in which they tried this. As a result, the pseudo-medical schools not only made no gains, but actually lost additional states due to scandals involving the alleged selling of diplomas in order to swell their ranks, the old-timers say.

What is certain is that a state-by-state legislative effort has been exerted by the CNME/AANP to not only license graduates of their schools, but to expressly *forbid* graduates of other schools to practice. The rationale for this is that CNME-schooled graduates are fully-trained physicians, while everyone else got a scanty education by mail or at the feet of an older naturopath. Legislators, on the lookout for anything that endangers the public health, have largely accepted this revisionist history.

As a result, the graduates of the aforementioned schools found themselves increasingly unable to be licensed. Trained either before any pseudo-medical schools existed, or before the CNME existed to "accredit" them, these naturopaths desired the freedom to practice; they were trained to practice as full-fledged healthcare providers in a non-medical mode, and now were being treated as though they never existed. In the New Order, they realized, there are only two citizens: the naturopathic physician who wants parity with the medical doctor, and the traditional naturopath, who generally opposes licensure as an affront to constitutional freedom.

> Legislators, on the lookout for anything that endangers the public health, have largely accepted this revisionist history.

As time has passed, this has become a moot point, as the aging classical naturopaths give up practice or die off. The very few remaining non-CNME schools do not have the facilities or resources to compete and cannot offer the breadth of training that the schools of yesteryear did.

> "Together with the increased use of technology in medicine, allopathic methodology rose while natural healing declined and **the last college offering a degree in naturopathic medicine, Western States Chiropractic College in Portland Oregon, closed its doors***. Still on the books in a few key states, licensing laws governing naturopathic doctors kept the door open for a renaissance in naturopathic medicine. In 1956 naturopathic doctors across the Northwest came together to found the National College of Naturopathic Medicine (NCNM) in Seattle, Washington. This marked the first bursts of the Naturopathic profession. The next thirty years would bring unprecedented growth as the role of primary-care professionals in the diagnosis and natural treatment of patients expanded and became the mainstay for naturopathic doctors. Two decades later graduates of the NCNM formed what would become Bastyr University in Seattle Washington in 1978 based upon the principles and inspiring example of Dr. John Bastyr, one of NCNM's founders. 1978 also brought NCNM to Portland Oregon where it has flourished for the past thirty years. Five medical schools currently hold accreditation by the Council on Naturopathic Medical Education (CNME). The CNME is the accrediting agency recognized by the U.S. Secretary of Education that grants accreditation to four-year medical programs leading to a doctoral degree in Naturopathic Medicine annotated as N.D. or N.M.D., which are considered synonymous."
>
> (from the web site of the Oregon State Board of Naturopathic Medicine)
>
> **The ongoing myth that is widely repeated: that the last naturopathic school was gone before the founding of NCNM. The fact is that other schools, which were not pseudo-medical, still existed. One by one, these have been forced out of existence.**

* Emphasis ours.

107

The popular explanation

for the disappearance of the old naturopathic schools and the dwindling supply of the practitioners themselves goes like this:

After World War II, life modernized at a rapid rate and scientific knowledge increased tremendously. With the development of antibiotics, vaccines, and other new classes of drugs, orthodox medicine was more effective than it ever was, and many of the health problems people used to consult drugless practitioners for were now easily cured by your family medical doctor.

The truth is a bit more complicated.

Pressure was exerted to increase educational requirements for naturopathic doctors (just as orthodox medicine had gradually converted all its schools from two-year to four-year programs). As in the case of the medical doctors, the numbers of naturopaths were reduced by the financial burden of schooling.

The other factor was legislation requiring an education in subjects pertinent to medical doctors but which had been heretofore considered irrelevant to naturopathic doctors. The "basic science" requirement for licensure was an issue of contention for an earlier generation of naturopaths, chiropractors, and other practitioners. The resurrection of this idea, and the enforcement of it, changed educational content and began to change naturopaths themselves.

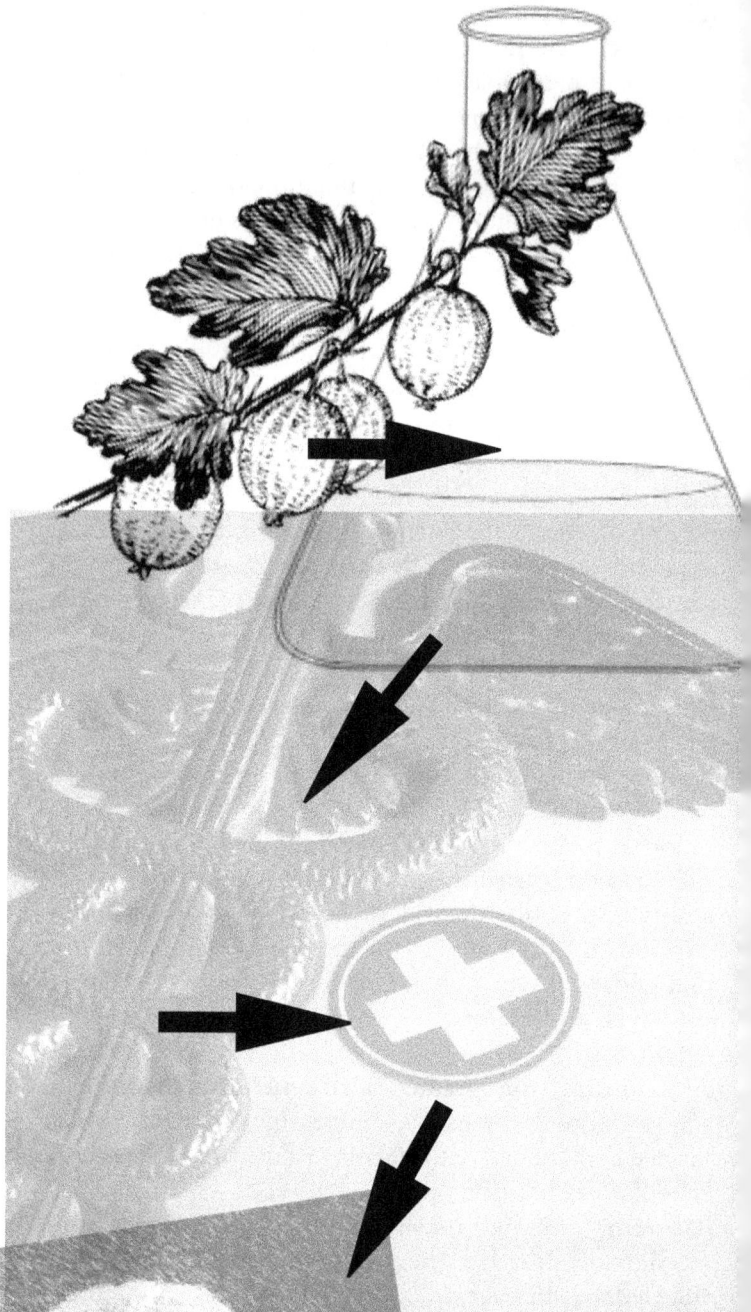

THE NEW NATUROPATHS

Basic Science Legislation
An Examination Into Its Origin, Purposes, and Effects
By Dr. R.A. Budden

The chief argument of the proponents of basic science legislation is that it is for the good of the people: that its sole purpose is to defend the public against incompetent doctors and charlatans.

If this argument can be sustained, it means that the organizations listed under "opponents", together with their vast following, are either blind to the public interest or are willfully careless of it.

Such a conclusion is preposterous. It must be apparent to the intelligent reader that the "opponents" are as sincere and successful in their care for the sick, and are as anxious for the public good and as ready to protect it against incompetents and charlatans as are the proponents.

It is clear that we must look [elsewhere] for the answer to the "why" of basic science legislation…

Investigation revealed an alarming fact. A questionnaire circulated by a great national magazine brought to light the surprising truth that more people showed allegiance to physiological and drugless methods than to purely medical treatments. Worse yet: the drugless world had developed its own schools and colleges; institutions of learning devoted exclusively to the teaching of the sciences peculiar to human therapeutics from the non-medical standpoint, well equipped and staffed by competent teachers.

The recoil from this situation gave rise in the minds of the medical chiefs to the idea of adverse legislation. It was apparent that if the drugless schools continued to flourish and to increase in value to the community and the country at large, it would be too late to attack them.

Thus the basic science idea was born. Drugless schools have no state endowments; they must depend on contributions from their alumni and upon tuition. If, then, their graduates could be compelled by law to face a medically minded examining board, their difficulties would be increased and their ambition inhibited. They might even be driven out of the field altogether.

Public health organizations are used to spread propaganda against the drugless physician. School and visiting nurses, charity associations, public clinics, industrial accident dispensaries, in fact everywhere that medical physicians are employed *in the public service*, there is a rostrum from which the anti-drugless bias is broadcast. Even in the medical schools themselves, mo matter whether they are maintained by public taxation, a special time is reserved for diatribes against drugless schools and practitioners. Great efforts are also put forth to keep non-medical physicians from occupying places on boards of health and other public offices…

It is certain also from the record that the passage of this legislation in other states had resulted in the closing of the colleges of drugless healing and that the extermination of this method of practice is within the realm of possibility…And whatever may be said with regard to the intent of the law, the result of its enactment is to ultimately leave the field of therapeutics clear of all competition to the medical men.

> **A questionnaire circulated by a great national magazine brought to light the surprising fact that more people showed allegiance to physiological and drugless methods than to purely medical treatments.**

(Dr. Budden was Dean of Western States Chiropractic College Naturopathic Program. Printed in *Naturopath and Herald of Health*, Jan. 1937, p. 26)

An interesting parallel with Dr. Budden's observation back in the 1930s would occur in the 1990s. The report by Eisenberg[*] that more Americans were visiting "alternative" healers than medical doctors opened up this old wound and was responsible for both the establishment of a Government office to oversee such practices (the Office of Complementary and Alternative Medicine) and the renewed battle for "turf" that has always characterized the struggle between "irregulars" and the medical orthodoxy.

The matter of required medical education was reduced to its simplest and most rational by Q. M. Cheatham, DC, ND:◆

> "The problems, field, and purpose of medicine DIFFER ENTIRELY from Chiropractic—and, therefore, its curriculum differs. When one considers that medicine attempts to cover everything from two seconds after conception to the very last breath of life—embracing drugs by the THOUSANDS—many of them exceedingly poisonous and dangerous—AND surgery, obstetrics, dermatology, exanthemata, and many other fields into which chiropractors as a body scarcely enter at all, it can be quickly seen that a chiropractor at the end of eighteen months is FAR BETTER fitted and trained for HIS FIELD and work than is a medical man for his practice in thirty-six months. And did you ever stop to think that a medical man gets only twice the training—thirty-six months—for perhaps twenty times as large and complicated a field?"

Most medical schools at the time were two-year or three-year courses with a year's residency requirement. A chiropractic education was correspondingly shorter. Both fields have since instituted a standard of four years' training, but the comparison and the points Dr. Cheatum makes still have validity, even if they are outdated.

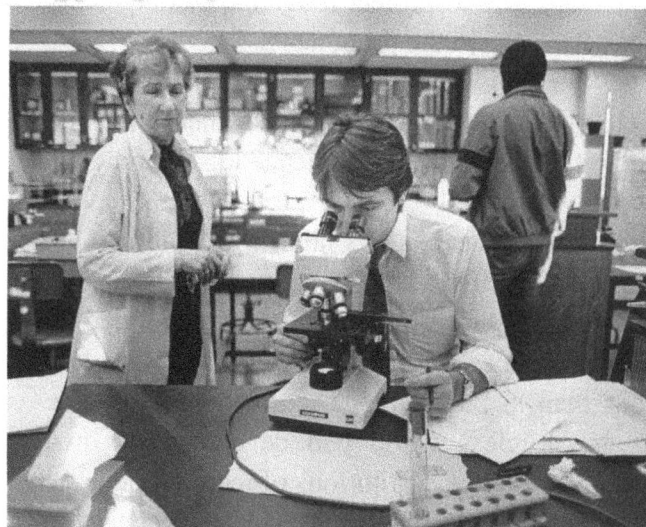

In this press photo from the September 17, 1985 edition of *The Seattle Times*, John Bastyr College of Naturopathic Medicine is before the public eye as an up-to-date, science-oriented institution. Working at the microscope is student Patrick Bufi, observed by Dr. Danile Keily. Photo by Greg Gilbert.

[*] Eisenberg, D.M., Kessler, R.C., Foster, C., et al: Unconventional Medicine in the United States. *N Engl J Med.* 1993: 328:246-252
◆ Q.M. Cheatham, ND; "How Long Should It Take To Make A Good Chiropractor?", *The Lighthouse,* Journal of the Nashville School of Drugless Therapy, 1937

110

1991—

- **Arno Koegler, ND, third president of the International Society of Naturopathic Physicians, dies.** He studied in his native Germany under Emanual Felke, whose expertise in Iridology and Homeopathy influenced Koegler's later practice. He would work as long as sixteen hours a day and saw an uncommonly large number of patients daily (as many as 200!). He taught at Canadian Memorial Chiropractic College in their naturopathic program. The founders of the later Ontario College of Naturopathic Medicine (now Canadian College of Naturopathic Medicine) were all trained by him.

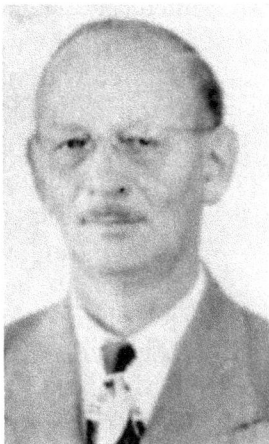

1992—

- **Southwest College of Naturopathic Medicine**, a pseudo-medical naturopathic school, opens in Scottsdale, Arizona. It is founded by Michael Cronin, Konrad Kail, Dana Keaton, Hugh Hawk, and Kyle Cronin. The professional title of NMD (Doctor of Naturopathic Medicine) was instituted by the Practice Act in this, the only state to specifically use that title (as an academic title, however, the NMD has existed since 1960 and has been offered by several schools—none of them CNME schools).

- **Veteran Arizona naturopaths** from the generation of Bernard Jensen and Paavo Airola find themselves increasingly unable to practice due to the new licensing law that favors the modern pseudo-medically trained naturopaths. The older NDs supported the new licensing bill after being told they would be "grandfathered" in, but were then excluded once the new board was in place.

- **Ontario College of Naturopathic Medicine changes its name** to Canadian College of Naturopathic Medicine.

- **On March 10, 1992, Donald Hayhurst, NMD, files a legal complaint** regarding a letter sent to the U.S. Secretary of Education by Randall Bradley, ND (then President of the Nebraska Association of Naturopathic Physicians). The letter allegedly libeled and slandered Hayhurst and attacked his credibility and background in the profession. However, under Nebraska law, such actions must be filed within one year. As the letter had been mailed March 10, 1990 and written almost a year earlier than that, the court decided against judgment against Bradley. Hayhurst said that he did not have access to the letter until the Department of Education finally responded to his repeated requests for the document. Nevertheless, the District Court found that the cause of action was time-barred (Hayhurst v. Bradley, No. 92-2826, United States Court of Appeals, Eighth Circuit).

1993—

- **The Oregon Senate passes a bill changing the legal wording** of "Naturopathy" to "Naturopathic Medicine" and removes the word "drugless" in the practice act. A trail blazer in this area is William Turska, ND, who objected to the term "drugless", saying "All therapeutic agents are drugs. Good drugs can become bad drugs and bad, good; it's all in how you use them."

- **AANP lobbyists succeed in a legislative effort** to have Washington State change its scope of practice for naturopaths, **allowing the prescribing of legend drugs, including**

> "In its modern day concept Naturopathic Medicine includes any physiological method which has been demonstrated to be clinically effective and conforms to the Naturopathic philosophy."
>
> --From Page 2 of the 1975 catalogue of the National College of Naturopathic Medicine, illustrating the intention to re-design the profession to include medical interventions.

> **Many modern naturopathic leaders have lamented the new direction, yet acknowledge the appeal to the contemporary naturopathic student in training that is supposedly "the equal of a medical doctor".**
>
> "This approach is increasingly referred to as "green allopathy." But the vast body of knowledge that naturopathic education presents in this arena makes such an approach seductive, especially in a culture that more or less expects, supports, reinforces, and pays for an 'allopathic' approach to diagnosis and treatment."
>
> (*Textbook of Natural Medicine*, Vol. 3, Chap. 3, A Hierarchy Of Healing: The Therapeutic Order, p. 37)

1994—

- **Harold Dick, ND dies.** Dick was a 1955 graduate of Western States College who did a three-year preceptorship with the legendary O.G. Carroll, who had encouraged him to become a naturopath. He established his own clinic in 1959 and continued using the highly effective Carroll protocol of constitutional hydrotherapy, dietary intolerance testing, and simple botanical compounds. He was an expert iridologist. He would go on to study acupuncture in the Far East; but he did not incorporate it into his practice, as he found that the methods he learned from Carroll were more effective♦.

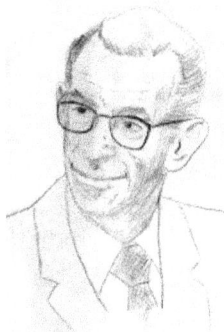

♦ A profound statement, since acupuncture is the most rigorously researched and documented alternative medicine methodology today.

He was openly critical of the latter-day naturopathic schools and their increasingly medical orientation. He felt, like Carroll before him, that **the emphasis on orthodox medical science was in itself unscientific, while the empirically-arrived-at and reliable low-tech methods he and other more traditional naturopaths used were far more scientific.** He was also a vocal opponent of synthetic vitamins and inorganic mineral supplements, which NDs had begun to use in abundance. He often said that they were "the most processed and dangerous drugs in the world."

Countless naturopathic students and established doctors made pilgrimages to his clinic to learn how he performed seeming miracles, and came away with profound changes in their thinking at the wonder of simple non-medical interventions.

His practice would be assumed by his daughter, Letitia Dick, ND.

- **John Bastyr College becomes Bastyr University of Natural Health Sciences.** In the same year, from the National Institutes of Health's Office of Alternative Medicine awards the school almost $1 million in research funds to research alternative therapies for patients with HIV and AIDS.

- **Central States College re-opens** in Columbus, Ohio. Known variously in the past as Central States College of Physiatrics and Central States College of Naturopathy, it re-opens under the name **Central States College of Health Sciences**. Robert McKinney and David Joseph, Jr. obtained the charter to Harry Riley Spitler's old school and re-established what was once one of the flagship schools in the U.S.

1995—

- **The NIH Office of Alternative Medicine** appointed an eleven-person panel to define and describe complementary and alternative medicine. The group was dominated by pseudo-medical naturopaths and traditional Chinese medicine practitioners. No chiropractors were appointed to the panel.

- The City Council of Seattle approves **the country's first federally-subsidized naturopathic clinic**, affiliated with Bastyr University.

- **John Bartholomew Bastyr, DC, ND, dies**. He was co-founder of National College of Naturopathic Medicine and namesake of the later Bastyr University.

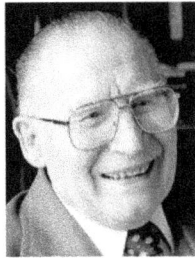

  Bastyr, a graduate of Seattle College of Chiropractic and Northwest Institute of Drugless Therapy, was a fixture in the Seattle area for over fifty years. He was inspired to go into the field by Dr. Harry Bonnelle, a naturopath who had written many articles published in *Naturopath and Herald of Health*. While a general practitioner, Bastyr excelled in obstetrics and delivered hundreds of babies. He once closed his office temporarily to work at the side of O.G. Carroll to learn the great naturopath's method of hydrotherapy. While Harold Dick and Leo Scott spent several *years* with Carroll, Bastyr was reputedly unhappy with the lack of orthodox science driving the man's practice, and spent only six months there.

  His insistence on adopting all methods from conventional medicine and science that would embellish Naturopathy made him the prototypical naturopath of the modern age, and the single person contemporary NDs are most modeled after.

- Canadian sociologist Heather Boon studied the educational curriculum and student experiences at **Canadian College of Naturopathic Medicine** during the 1993-1994 academic year. Her findings, published in 1995, show that the first two years concentrated on standard allopathic biomedical science courses, with only introductory naturopathic subjects addressed the second year. Courses in naturopathic modalities required during the third year were considered by much of the student body to be overly medicalized. Fourth year, as elsewhere, clinical training was emphasized and this also had an allopathic slant. Boon reported that the CCNM students complained to the administration that **their training was not sufficiently naturopathic.**[*]

1996—

- **Maine, Vermont, and Utah all begin licensing** naturopathic physicians.

- In Minnesota, where naturopaths are not licensed, **Helen Healy, ND, is served with a cease-and-desist injunction**. As one of the new generation of naturopathic physicians who consider themselves primary care physicians, she unabashedly diagnosed and prescribed for patients, and was charged with practicing medicine without a license.

- **The Consortium of Naturopathic Medical Colleges** (later to be known as the American Association of Naturopathic Medical Colleges) begins the development of a standardized curriculum for all schools. That current generation of practitioners is largely unaware that this has already been established, in 1922 (The Associated Naturopathic Schools and Colleges of America—"ANSCA"). But the new regulating agency insists on a pseudo-medical curriculum for all schools, requiring a premedical education and including biomedical courses that were not considered part of naturopathic training before that time. **Schools not following this trend will not be considered for accreditation by the Council for Naturopathic Medical Education (CNME).**

- **Clyde Jensen**, holding a PhD in pharmacology, is appointed President of National College of Naturopathic Medicine. He will be the first in a series of non-ND administrators with knowledge and experience in the expansion of medical institutions.

---

[*] Boon, Heather. The Making of a Naturopathic Practitioner: The Education of Alternative Practitioners; *Health and Canadian Society* 3(1/2):15-41

1997—

- **University of Bridgeport**, Connecticut, begins its naturopathic program, bringing the number of pseudo-medical naturopathic schools in the U.S. to four. James Sensenig, ND, is founding Dean. A chiropractic program also resides at Bridgeport. The University is a private institution that was taken over by Rev. Sun Myung Moon's Unification Church with a $50 million grant that gave the church control of the board. It is the only University in the country that operates a chiropractic school.

- **John Thomas College of Naturopathic Medicine** opens in St. Charles, Missouri. It is a private postdoctoral training facility for MDs, DOs, and DCs who wish to become credentialed as naturopaths. They award the NMD degree after 27 months of didactic study and clinical internship in natural medicine at a pace that allows practicing physicians to maintain their practices at the same time. Regional outpatient clinics and hospitals for in-patient training are affiliated with JTC in Missouri, New York, Florida, Idaho, Texas, Arizona, and California.

  While JTC is accredited by the Missouri Department of Higher Education, the Council for Naturopathic Medical Education (CNME), overseer of the pseudo-medical naturopathic schools, does not recognize John Thomas.

- **A class action suit is filed in Portland, Oregon in January against NCNM, AANP, and CNME**, alleging fraud and deceit in that the literature and marketing of the school, national association, and accrediting agency all knowingly mislead students as to the ability of the graduates to be recognized nationally as "primary care providers"

1998—

- **Scandal strikes Southwest College of Naturopathic Medicine in Arizona as the faculty is exposed for improprieties involving national board exam questions. The school's bank accounts are temporarily frozen and several officials are fired. Michael Cronin, ND steps down as President.**[*]

[*] Fehr-Snyder, K. "Naturopathic board director on leave". Arizona Republic, May 11, 2001; Naturopathic Board votes to fire chief: Allegations tied to credentials, paper shredding. *Arizona Republic*, May 12, 2001.

1999—

- **U.S. Secretary of Education Richard Riley denies the renewal of recognition** of the Council on Naturopathic Medical Education due to Southwest scandal, for not rescinding accreditation of the school.[♦]

- Legislative efforts on the part of National College of Naturopathic Medicine (Portland) and Bastyr University (Seattle) **attempted to gain the legal right for their graduates to inject narcotics in both Oregon and Washington** states. The legislatures of both states refused.

2000–

- **Arizona Auditor General found that the Arizona Naturopathic Physicians Examining Board had consistently adjusted applicants' exam scores** so that everyone taking the exam since 1998 had passed. In 1999, when 9 out of 18 scores were still too low, further adjustments were made. Inadequate record keeping and inattention to complaints by the board were noted by the Auditor General. [*]

  The Arizona Naturopathic Physicians Board of Medical Examiners made an admission that underplayed the seriousness of the situation: "The Board has not shown that its three-part examination was developed, scored, and maintained appropriately, which raises questions about whether it can be used to measure licensing applicants' competency to practice Naturopathy. The Board also has not maintained adequate records to show that all licensed naturopaths have taken all required parts of the examination." (Report #00-9, June 2000)

2000–

- **The AANP sues the ANMA** (American Naturopathic Medical Association) and its founder, Dr. Don Hayhurst; the suit is dismissed in U.S. District Court in New Hampshire. Hayhurst had taken legal action to prevent restrictive licensing laws favoring pseudo-medical NDs being passed.

-

[♦] Davenport, D.K. *Performance Audit: Arizona Naturopathic Physicians Board of Medical Examiners*. Report No. 00-9, June 2000.
[*] *Ibid.*

- Increasingly, bills introduced by AANP lobbyists specifically prevent traditional and classical naturopaths from practicing. Hayhurst has been a dogged opponent of such protectionism, and earned the enmity of the pseudo-medicalist camp.♦

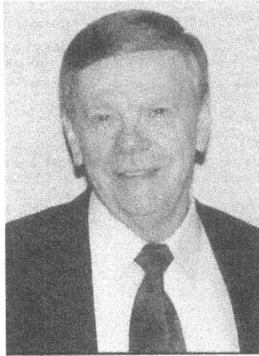

Donald C. Hayhurst, ND

- **Boucher Institute of Naturopathic Medicine** opens in British Columbia, Canada. Named for Joe Boucher, co-founder of National College of Naturopathic medicine, it is another pseudo-medical school that quickly is awarded candidacy for CNME accreditation, allowing Boucher's graduates to sit for the NPLEX licensing examination in the U.S.

> **"Insufficiently trained providers may actually be a threat to public safety."**
> **--Andrew Rubman, ND**
> (in reference to non-CNME schools, at the White House Commission on Complementary and Alternative Medical Services, Dec. 5, 2000)

- **The West Coast Naturopathic School in Vancouver, B.C. opens**. Unlike Boucher Institute, this school is not approved by the Canadian Department of Education that recognizes the pseudo-medical schools. It is also excluded from candidacy for accreditation by the CNME, so its graduates will not be eligible to sit for the NPLEX licensing exam[*].

- **The Council on Naturopathic Medical Education (CNME) loses recognition by the U.S. Department of Education and the National Advisory Committee on Institutional Quality and Integrity (NACIQI), due to scandals in Arizona.** The National Advisory Committee voted to deny The Council on Naturopathic Medical Education (CNME) recognition as an accrediting agency citing numerous compromises of the CNME's own written standards. (Decision of Secretary Richard W. Riley, Docket No. 00-06-0, DoEd Accrediting Agency Recognition Proceeding, January 16, 2001).[*]

- In May 2001, the **Arizona Naturopathic Physicians Board of Medical Examiners executive director is fired** following allegations that he shredded documents, copied exams, and misrepresented his credentials.[*]

- **Dennis Robbins, PhD, MPH**, assumes the presidency of National College of Naturopathic Medicine.

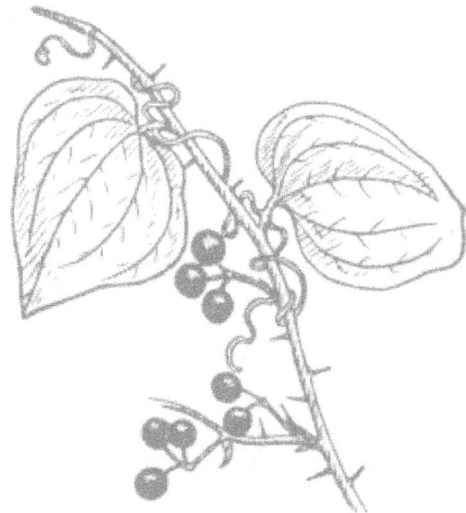

[*] Barrett, Stephen (2003-06-13). "Naturopathic Accreditation Agency Loses Federal Recognition - But Reapproval Seems Likely". Quackwatch. http://www.quackwatch.org/01QuackeryRelatedTopics/Naturopathy/accreditation.html. Retrieved 2009-04-17.

[*] Fehr-Snyder, K. "Naturopathic board director on leave". Arizona Republic, May 11, 2001. Naturopathic Board votes to votes to fire chief: Allegations tied to credentials, paper shredding. Arizona Republic, May 12, 2001.

♦ American Naturopathic Medical Association web site

[*] Nine private naturopathic schools in Canada are considered "substandard" by the pseudo-medical schools and are seen as a threat to the modern naturopathic physician's livelihood.

- **Bernard Jensen, DC, ND, dies** on February 22, a month before his 93rd birthday. One of the most well-known classical naturopaths in the country, he had received an overwhelming number of awards and honoraria, but by this time was *persona non grata* in the eyes of the upcoming pseudo-medical naturopathic community, as were most of his generation.

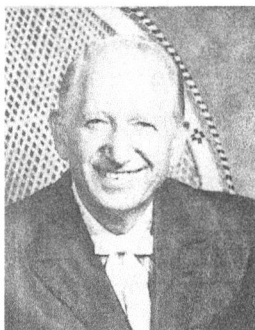

Jensen was expert in a wide variety of naturopathic modalities, including hydrotherapy, colon therapy, fasting, reflexology, botanical medicine, nutrition, and even acupuncture. An inveterate learner, he was estimated to have accumulated over 6000 hours of postgraduate instruction. He traveled to sixty-five countries in the course of his studies, and was once received by the Dalai Lama.

For decades he operated the Hidden Valley Health Ranch in Escondido, California, which offered residential detoxification programs, fasting, hydrotherapy, and other procedures, and which provided 60% of its food from its own organic gardens. He treated over 350,000 patients.

Dr. Jensen was possibly best known for his contributions to the field of iris diagnosis, and was probably the foremost authority in America on the subject. His textbook, *The Science and Practice of Iridology*, remains a classic of its kind. He wrote more than 40 books, including *Tissue Cleansing Through Bowel Management, Chemistry of Man,* and *Foods That Heal.*

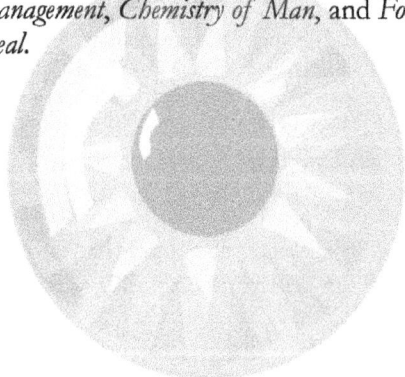

- **Animosity continues to build** between the pseudo-medical naturopaths (called "green allopaths" by their critics) and traditional naturopaths who emphasize detoxification and diet (called "weeder-seeders" by the others).

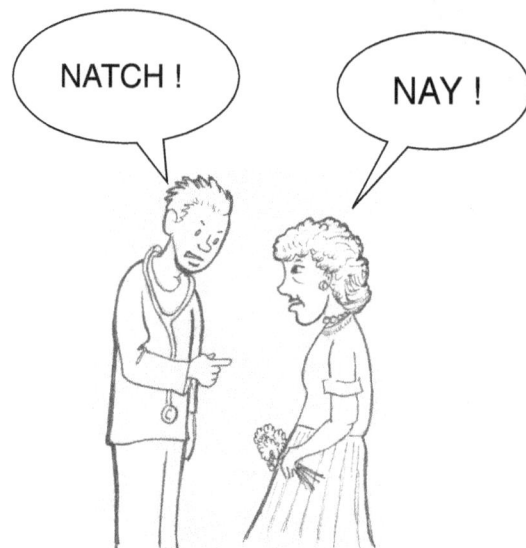

NDs had historically referred to themselves as naturopaths (NAY-cher-o-paths), but increasingly, the new generation began to pronounce it NAT-cher-o-paths, creating yet another distinction between the two groups. Although dictionaries have long supported the first pronunciation, the latter has gained popularity. Is it a long "A" because it is based on nature, or is it a short "A" because it's "natural"?

- The Florida Naturopathic Physicians Association (FNPA) submits **legislative efforts to re-establish naturopathic licensure in Florida.** This group, representing a broad spectrum of naturopaths, sought to reinstate the (purely naturopathic) scope of practice now enjoyed by only the seven survivors of the abolishment of the license in 1957. The bill dies in committee. In the same year, the Florida Association of Naturopathic Medicine (FANM) introduces *their* bill, which includes the right to prescribe drugs and perform surgery. The organization, affiliated with the national AANP, also demanded equal rights and hospital privileges as medical doctors. Not surprisingly, this bill also dies in committee.

- **Bastyr University receives its first million-dollar individual gift** from Stephen Bing of Los Angeles.

2002–

The Bastyr University bookstore carries a reprint of Henry Lindlahr's *Nature Cure*, with the explanatory remark "Dr. Lindlahr was the founder of American Naturopathy and introduced the United States to the German Nature Cure movement."

History is being revised once again. Benedict Lust is no longer the founder, according to Bastyr University. Lindlahr now wears the crown, perhaps because of his reputation as the one who put Naturopathy on "scientific footing"?

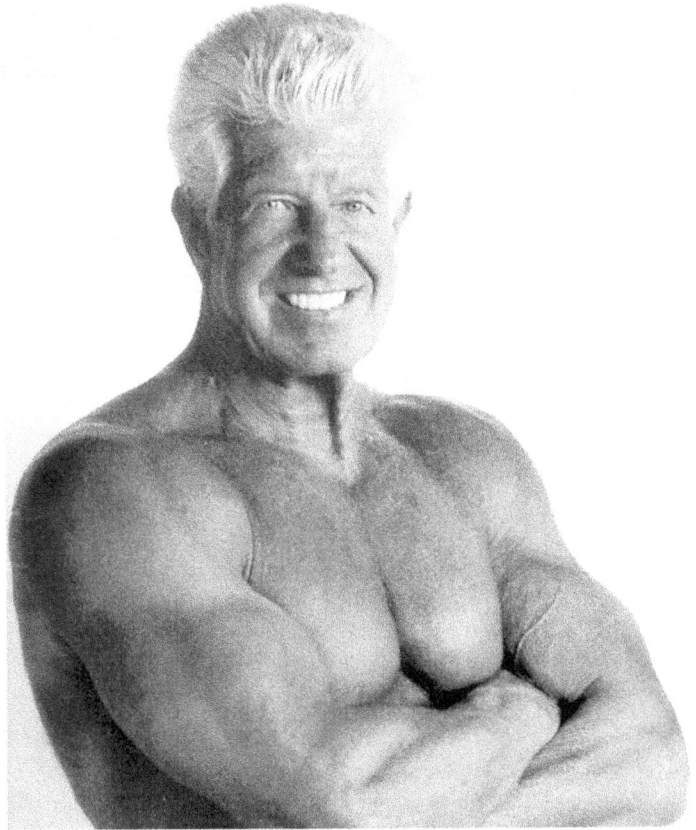

2003–

- **G. E. Poesnecker, ND, dies.** Long the director of the Clymer Clinic and later the Clymer Healing Research Center of Pennsylvania, Poesnecker was the author of *It's Only Natural*, and he republished Lindlahr's classic *Nature Cure* with modern commentary in the year 2000.

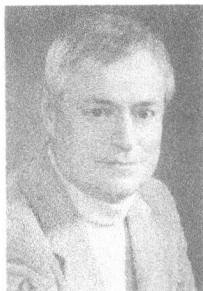

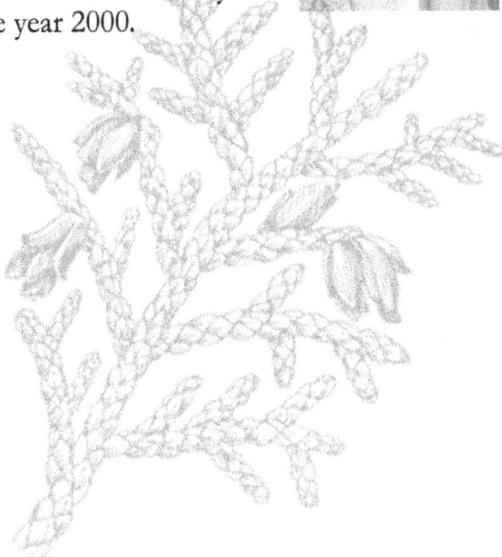

Bob Delmonteque, ND, pictured above at the incredible age of 84, is an example of an earlier generation of traditional naturopaths for whom teaching health was the professional goal, rather than diagnosing and treating illness.

Like Paul Bragg, the Malibu naturopath has served for decades as one of Hollywood's top health experts and celebrity trainers. Before the term "wellness" was even coined, Delmonteque was sharing his regimen of seven basic elements: proper exercise, healthy diet, spiritual thinking, rest and recuperation, pure water, sunshine, and fresh air.

Also like Bernarr Macfadden and Jesse Mercer Gehman, he has been an avid bodybuilder all his life and trained a number of famous athletes such as Rocky Marciano, boxing's only undefeated heavyweight champion. He even assisted the first astronaut, Alan Shepherd, in his fitness program. Born in 1919, he became involved in early longevity research *back in the late 1940s*. The concept of anti-aging medicine is generally thought to be a recent one, but Delmonteque and his colleagues were far ahead of the curve. This 2003 portrait of "Dr. Bob" above is all the evidence one needs.

117

In 2003, the Council on Naturopathic Medical Education (CNME), the accreditation body for pseudo-medical schools, regains recognition by the U.S. Department of Education.

ACCREDITED?

such as record keeping, physical assets, financial status, makeup of the governing body, catalogue characteristics, nondiscrimination policy, and self-evaluation system..." *

Up until this year, non-CNME school graduates have been certified by the American Naturopathic Medical Certification and Accreditation Board (ANMCAB). This group is dissolved in 2003, and was replaced by separate bodies:

1) The American Naturopathic Certification Board (ANCB), for certifying what are now called traditional naturopaths;

2) The American Naturopathic Medical Accreditation Board (ANMAB) for certifying those who have graduated from an accredited medical program and have training and experience approved by the Board (as well as examination), which will lead to board certification as a naturopathic physician. ANMAB also provides board certification for naturopathic doctors and traditional naturopaths who come from approved schools (and who still must pass an examination by ANMAB).

ANMAB is registered with the Department of Consumer and Regulatory Affairs in Washington, D.C.

What are the differences among the certifying bodies?

The casual observer (but also the average student at a CNME-accredited school) misses a vital point: Accreditation for naturopathic programs is an entirely voluntary process. Accreditation of an educational program by a board simply validates that the program has been thoroughly investigated and recognized as worthy. The investigation is conducted by a qualified group of people familiar with the programs offered. Also, the programs are evaluated for their financial stability, so as to protect the interests of students.

ANCB and ANMAB have standards that hark back to the days of the National Board of Naturopathic Examiners (est. 1940) for the competence of the applicants, and the Associated Naturopathic Schools and Colleges of America (est. 1922) for the quality of the educational programs.

The CNME, however, thought to do what no one ever felt the need to do: petition the United States Department of Education for recognition. This official government acknowledgment is the linchpin of the pseudo-medical naturopaths' claims to respectability. Yet, unlike other accrediting panels that evaluate the aptitude of faculty members and the quality of the curriculum, the CNME is centered on "factors

It would surprise many, if not most, students at the five pseudo-medical schools that **the Federal Government does not accredit educational institutions or programs of any kind, according to the United States Department of Education (DoEd).** Because the U.S. does not have a centralized authority to accredit and regulate educational providers, school accreditation in this country is a completely voluntary process. Accreditation is granted by private, non-profit, independent, non-governmental organizations (NGOs). No accreditation authority actually exists at the federal, state and local levels of government. In the United States, degree-granting authority of a school is up to the individual state where it is charted. Federal accreditation is not required. At this point, there are six schools that have legal authority from their state to grant naturopathic degrees, yet pseudo-medical naturopaths constantly claim that only *their* schools are "accredited".

The true advantage of recognition by the U.S. Department of Education is in "Title 7"—providing access to educational loans for naturopathic students. The CNME schools could now swell their ranks by making it easier to attend their colleges. Naturopathic students never qualified for loans before. The CNME schools gained more students, gained more "clout" with lending institutions for those increasing numbers, and they gained increased respectability from their "recognition" by a Federal agency. This last aspect they have adopted as major evidence of superiority.

The professional profile of Joseph E. Pizzorno, Jr., president emeritus of Bastyr University, makes this claim:

> "When Dr. Pizzorno co-founded Bastyr, no mechanism existed to objectively establish credibility for schools of natural medicine. In response, he helped established the pathway to accreditation...As part of his long-standing effort to establish scientific standards for natural medicine education, Dr. Pizzorno co-founded the Council for Naturopathic Medical Education (CNME) in 1978. He wrote the standards and spearheaded CNME's successful effort to secure accreditation from the U.S. Department of Education in 1987."

* Raso, J., *"Alternative" Healthcare: A Complete Guide,* 1994 Prometheus Books, p. 104

California licenses naturopaths again. The California Association of Naturopathic Physicians (CANP), a pseudo-medical membership organization, had been unsuccessful in several previous attempts to introduce licensing bills. Whenever bills were amended by committees to include traditional naturopaths already practicing in the state, the CANP would retract their own bill.

A meeting of the two naturopathic camps to find a mutually acceptable solution was fruitless. California Naturopathic Association president Dr. Angela Burr-Madsen, and Dr. Robert Thiel, president of the California State Naturopathic Medical Association, both representing the traditional naturopaths, met with Dr. Sally LeMont of the CANP and with legislators. The traditional naturopathic community (many times larger than the 50 members of CANP) agreed to embrace the pseudo-medical educational standards in insisting on seven years' education, a clinical internship in a naturopathic facility, and national board certification by a specifically naturopathic exam. Both the CNA and CANP would have input into the standards. Also, the amended bill would allow NDs to bill insurance, act as primary care practitioners, and have hospital privileges, as the pseudo-medical naturopaths wanted. Practitioners who did not meet the standards would be able to practice in an educational mode, but would not be able to call themselves "naturopathic doctor" or "naturopathic physician". The proposed bill would be non-discriminatory and recognize both types of naturopaths, and would restrain CANP from engaging in further discriminatory licensing bills.

Dr. LeMont, speaking for CANP, flatly refused.

The CANP, as an arm of the American Association of Naturopathic Physicians (AANP), wanted nothing less than the right of their members to use prescription drugs and perform surgery, and objected to part of the proposed bill that would limit them to traditional naturopathic modalities. Their all-or-nothing philosophy was not about to change.

In 2003, a new bill (SB 907) was introduced by Senate president Pro Tem John Burton. It would prohibit anyone from being licensed unless he or she was a graduate of a CNME-accredited school; in other words, a pseudo-medical naturopath. When traditional naturopaths complained about the exclusionary nature of the license, Burton threatened to repeal business and professional codes that allowed traditional naturopaths to practice without being subject to charges of practicing medicine.

Conventional doctors of the California Medical Association, which had previously fought naturopathic bills, met behind closed doors with the CANP and together amended the bill to insure that NDs would not call themselves "physicians", and that their medicinal formulary was under the oversight of the Boards of medicine and Pharmacy.

The naturopathic formulary for California includes hormones and prescription drugs as well as herbal medicines and vitamins. The text read: "A naturopathic doctor may prescribe natural and synthetic hormones, local anesthetics, and epinephrine and furnish other prescription drugs consistently with the scope and supervision requirements of a person licensed as a nurse practitioner". The pseudo-medical naturopaths relinquished their desire to be called "primary care providers" in order to be licensed. The bill refers to B&P code 2836, which deals with "categories of nurse practitioners and standards for nurses to hold themselves out as nurse practitioners in each category." The "naturopathic physicians", as they prefer to be called, actually have the medicolegal status of nurses. A traditional naturopath is still allowed to practice, but cannot call himself or herself "ND" or "Doctor of Naturopathy", but simply "naturopath".

The biggest push to make this bill a law came from Stephen Bing, celebrity, movie producer, media mogul, and contributor to many political campaigns. A supporter of pseudo-medical naturopathic care, he donated $1 million to Bastyr University, and it is speculated that he underwrote many of the costs of legislative efforts in California such as this bill. As a result of whatever financing they received, Bastyr hired top lobbying firm Advocation, Inc. to push the bill through the legislature.

The *Sacramento Bee* reported, "And, as with all medical turf battles, whether SB 907 lives or dies has everything to do with politics and nothing to do with whether it enhances or imperils the health of Californians." ♦

Dr. Robert Thiel, then president of the California State Naturopathic Medical Association, interpreted the law as the beginning of medical control of the entire country's natural health industry: "How can a
(Continued)

♦ Walters, Dan. "Naturopathic Bill Moves With Push From Movie Tycoon". *Sacramento Bee*. June 30, 2003

California naturopathic licensing bill betray the natural health movement? California is a national trend-setter. By allowing medical doctors and pharmacists (professions that by definition are not part of natural health movement) to influence dietary supplements, SB 907 is setting the stage for medical control of the dietary supplement industry".

Already in 2003, The *Journal of the American Medical Association* went on record* as saying that "If dietary supplements have or promote…biological activity, they should be considered as active drugs". On that same day Sen. Richard Durbin of Illinois introduced SB-722, a bill that would restrict dietary supplements, or put them under medical control under the banner of "public safety".

2005–

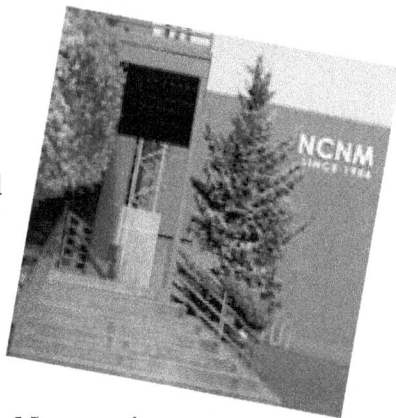

- **National College of Naturopathic Medicine** changes its name to National College of *Natural* Medicine.

- **The Arizona Board of Naturopathic Medicine lists its disciplinary actions** in its web site. Between December 2000 and July 2006 the Board took thirty disciplinary actions against twenty-six licensed naturopaths. Only three of the actions were for a benign reason: failure to maintain adequate continuing educational requirements. The other 27 were for more substantial infractions that could or did result in harm to the public.

- **Florida lobbyists again introduce a restrictive licensing bill** that will prevent anyone other than graduates of CNME schools to practice if licensure is reinstated. H1261 and S2678 fail to restore licensure to the State of Florida.

In the October 2005 issue of the *ANMA Monitor*, the online journal of the American Naturopathic Medical Association, this editorial from the office of the President sums up the divide between pseudo-medical naturopaths and traditional naturopaths, as well as the differences between the AANP and the ANMA:

This year things have gone very well and we can hope they're getting better. ANMA still holds true to its original beliefs: The root of the word Naturopath is NATURE! Some Naturopaths think that they should do their best to impersonate allopaths (M.D.'s). Drugs and surgery aren't natural. Invasive treatments are not what Hypocrites was after. He treated virtually all his patients with every known malady of the day with natural substances and natural methods…ANMA does not think Hypocrites would approve of Naturopaths doing breast implants and vasectomies, or performing abortions. ANMA supports or opposes legislation according to its original beliefs. These beliefs were adopted by you and your peers.

The ANMA, America's largest professional association for naturopathic practitioners, and the only such association recognized by the World Organization for Alternative Medicine, has been a driving force in the quest to restore natural medicine as a viable choice in Health care. ANMA has always been an organization of inclusion, welcoming doctors from all disciplines and all schools, providing they practice natural methods and do so within the laws of their state.

* *JAMA*, Mar. 23, 2003

Those who attend any of the CNME-accredited schools are told from the first day that they are getting a first-rate education and that no less an authority than the United States Government says so! A second sentiment that is nurtured is that anyone undergoing such a rigorous and comprehensive education should feel outrage that there are other types of naturopaths who assume the ND title without undergoing the same training as them.

An ongoing lament of graduates of the CNME-accredited pseudo-medical schools goes something like this: "Poorly-trained graduates of non-accredited programs and correspondence schools, who also claim the ND degree, put the public at risk."

Yet, Clayton College of Natural Health♦ (inarguably the most verbally attacked institution by the CNME) has these standards for its graduates:

- They must "provide a written and verbal description of services offered to each client."
- They must "specifically state that the consulting sessions are for educational purposes only, and that they do not diagnose, prescribe, cure or treat illnesses."
- They must "explain that a naturopathic consultant educates the client regarding natural approaches to health and improving his or her daily lifestyle choices."
- They must "Use only educational language with the client and on any written reports, forms, or notes."
- They must "strive to consistently empower the client to learn more about his/her own health, how to improve his/her daily living choices to be healthier and how to approach unhealthy conditions in a positive and natural way."
- A graduate should "refer to oneself as a consultant, and insure that all business cards, letterhead, brochures, etc. reflect the services provided."
- "Know your state and local laws, particularly those pertaining to dietary/nutrition and medical/healthcare scopes of practice."

Many feel that the hatred toward Clayton's program on the part of the CNME-approved institutions is a distraction: While creating the impression that the distance-learning students of the Clayton school are the major competitors of the pseudo-medical naturopaths, it obscures the knowledge that other schools (some with resident training) still exist and in some cases, exceed the CNME schools in naturopathic courses.

So what is so offensive about a naturopath who clearly claims to NOT be a physician, one who does not diagnose or prescribe or treat illness? The picture one gets from a pseudo-medical naturopath is that such people as the above are preying on the ignorance of the public and are woefully deficient in knowledge and ability.

Because traditional naturopaths do not practice medicine, diagnose or prescribe, perform invasive procedures, etc., the medical courses that the CNME curricula are weighted down with are not (and really should not be) imposed on them. When the apples-to-oranges comparison is halted, one sees that the number of *naturopathic* courses that non-CNME students take greatly outnumber those that the pseudo-medical NDs are required to take. Canyon College of California, for example, requires *double* the number of hours in naturopathic theory and practice than National College of Natural Medicine.

Bridge programs and postdoctoral institutions such as John Thomas College of Naturopathic Medicine never come up in these discussions of accredited schools vs. everyone else. How much of a danger would an already credentialed MD or DO, who then becomes a naturopath, pose to the public?

The Federal Government does not accredit educational institutions or programs of any kind, according to the United States Department of Education (DoEd).

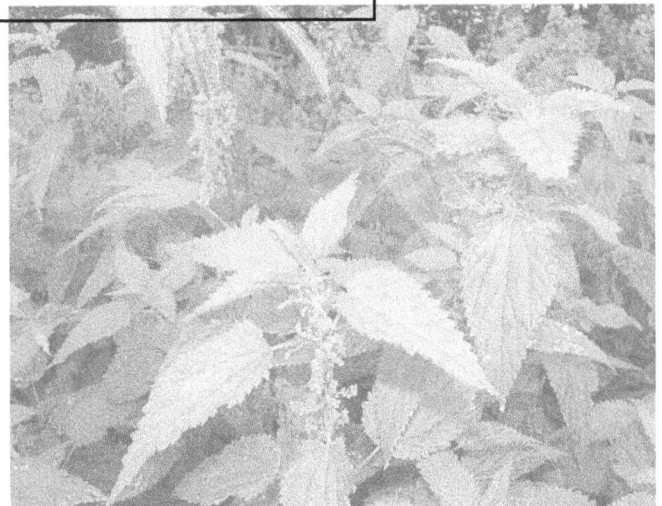

♦ Not to be confused with Clayton University of St. Louis, another school of natural medicine which closed in 1989. Its prestigious Board of Directors included pioneers and experts such as Nobel Prize winner Linus Pauling.

2003–

- After lobbying by the AANP, **the District of Columbia changes the longstanding licensing of naturopaths** to "registration", and enacts licensing of pseudo-medical naturopaths. The two-tier system recognizes "naturopaths" and "naturopathic physicians".

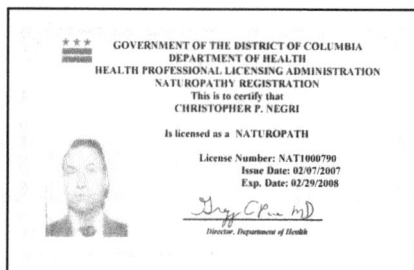

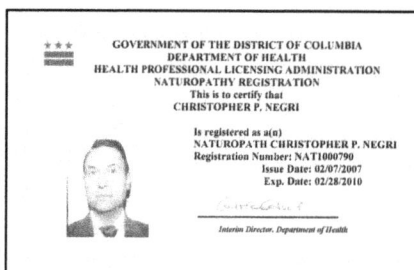

DC license before and after "licensed" becomes "registered".

- **Florida licensing failure.** After repeated legislative attempts by both traditional naturopaths and pseudo-medical naturopaths to reinstate licensing in Florida, the state decides to not license, stating that the scope of practice wanted by the pseudo-medical group was too broad, and that such a law would exclude traditional naturopaths and other types of practitioners from doing non-invasive health counseling, which does not require a license.

- **The Canadian Association of Naturopathic Doctors** (CAND) initiates a first-ever television campaign to promote naturopathic medicine, to enlist the public in demanding that they be included in the Regulated Health Professions Act, and to distinguish themselves from the traditional naturopaths (who are no less recognized by the government).

2005–

- **Bastyr University purchases a new campus** in a secluded spot in Kenmore, Washington, north of Seattle, for $12 million.

- **Central States College of Health Sciences in Columbus, Ohio also moves.** This reincarnation of Harry Riley Spitler's school of the 1940s will now share space with Columbus Community Hospital. The conventional medical setting arouses the interest of the

CNME, whose representatives visit and discuss candidacy for accreditation for the school. Robert McKinney, ND, President of Central States, is a prime mover in lobbying for naturopathic licensure in Ohio.

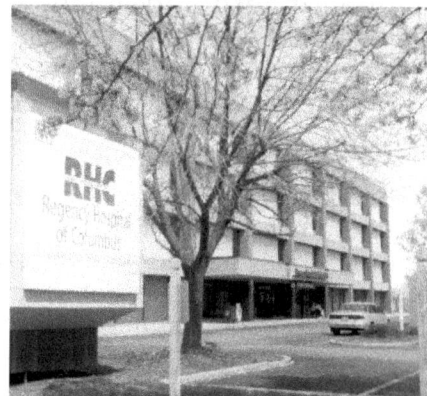

Central States College

While initially assisted by representatives from the CNME and the AANP, support for McKinney's efforts is suddenly retracted when talking with legislators, with the visitors insisting on exclusive licensing for their (pseudo-medical) graduates. Legislators dismiss the matter due to a divided profession. Central States, with a charter to issue degrees, finds itself in increasingly difficult circumstances. Instate graduates cannot be licensed, and licensable states, dominated by the CNME, shun their graduates. Central States alumni have nowhere to go.

- **Another try in Florida.** Bill H695 is introduced in Florida by the AANP affiliate group there, with wording that grants exclusive rights to practice to only pseudo-medical naturopaths. The bill does not make it through the Senate.

- *Naturopathic Doctor News and Review,* an online journal, debuts in August 2005.

- **National College of Naturopathic Medicine** changes its name to National College of *Natural* Medicine.

- **The Arizona Board of Naturopathic Medicine lists its disciplinary actions** in its web site. Between December 2000 and July 2006 the Board took thirty disciplinary actions against twenty-six licensed naturopaths. Only three of the actions were for a benign reason: failure to maintain adequate continuing educational requirements. The other 27 were for more substantial infractions that could or did result in harm to the public.

BUT WHERE'S THE MONEY COMING FROM?

A curious similarity to the history of the conventional allopathic medical field exists in the new naturopathic world. Back in the early 20th Century, when the allopaths were facing tough competition from osteopaths, homeopaths, eclectics, physio-medicalists, Thomsonians, and then naturopaths and chiropractors, they developed a new business plan. Funded by a small number of pharmaceutical companies that made the new synthetic drugs developed in Germany, the allopathic doctors implemented their plan to drive out all the other practitioners. United by the American Medical Association, they first adjusted their image. They were to be known far and wide as the most up to date, *scientific* doctors. Their schools were endowed with the finest equipment. They developed the most advanced life-saving surgery. They utilized the purest medicines—no crude plant extracts like the other doctors had used. These drugs were so potent and effective that you needed a prescription from an MD to get them!

But it was the lobbying of state medical boards to disallow graduates of non-allopathic schools to sit for licensure exams that really started to make the other practitioners disappear. With the stated goal of "improving medical education", it was easy to make those institutions that differed in philosophy lose their funding—just give them a poor rating. In a short time, 17 of 22 homeopathic medical colleges closed, all the physio-medicalist schools, and all but one of the eclectic colleges. Eventually, they would all disappear.

Ask almost anyone today who they think runs the medical field and they will answer: *pharmaceutical companies.*

A disturbing parallel exists with the rise and dominance of the pseudo-medical naturopaths. Under the lofty goal of improved education, they have (like the allopaths a century before) made their medical education require more money, more years, and more courses that have little to do with the practice of effective natural therapy. The very population set attracted to the schools has thus been changed. And the students of this new naturopathic medicine are taught to prescribe items the older NDs would never have touched: synthetic vitamin analogs and isolates, standardized extracts (not the whole herbal medicine), even prescription drugs. They increasingly veer away from tried-and-true naturopathic modalities in favor of methods that have been deemed "evidence-based". Only 2% of the new NDs are reputed to use joint manipulation in their practices, for example. A naturopath without manual therapies?

Like the allopaths before them, there has been an aggressive lobbying of state legislatures by these naturopaths to not simply license their practice, but to *exclude* other types of naturopaths and restrict even the use of the term "naturopathic doctor".

One might ask just *how* the pseudo-medical naturopathic colleges went from two to seven schools in North America in such a short time, or how the original flagship schools went from being small institutions to having large campuses. How did these schools create facilities that they can claim to be the equal of conventional medical training centers?

The emergence of the "nutraceutical"—a product that is based on a nutritional substance but acts correctively on unhealthy conditions like a medicine—is likely a part of the answer. Vitamins, herbs, amino acids, enzymes—all these substances and more can be combined to produce an original (and proprietary) product. The makers of these products endow the modern schools, and the modern NDs prescribe them.

PREPARE FOR YOUR FUTURE
IN THE HEALING ARTS FIELD

INVESTIGATE
NATUROPATHIC MEDICINE
OPPORTUNITIES UNLIMITED IN THIS
FASCINATING PROFESSION
Two Years College and Four Years
In Professional College Required
For Information About
THE NATIONAL COLLEGE OF
NATUROPATHIC MEDICINE
WRITE
1920 N. KILPATRICK, PORTLAND, OREGON

National College of Naturopathic Medicine occupied just part of a commercial building when this 1963 ad appeared.

In 1993, the third of the new pseudo-medical naturopathic schools opened in Arizona, propelled by a $500,000 first donation from a natural products company. Other such companies came forth also to fund the Southwest College of Naturopathic Medicine*, and this has become the model for new school development. As a result, the content of these new schools' programs focus on information based on industry funding—a radical change from the empirical findings preserved and taught by the more traditional naturopathic schools.

According to National College of Natural Medicine's 2010 ND Alumni Survey, 22.4% of their graduates "are employed by or are contracted with a nutraceutical company."

One might also ask why the nutraceutical companies were willing to produce product lines for such a small number of practitioners and how they were able to amass enough money as to lend so much financial support to these schools (and to fund political lobbying). Some speculate that these companies are themselves funded by invisible partners—conventional pharmaceutical companies.

Makers of Botanical Medicines Acquired by
International Pharmaceutical Companies

Natural Medicine Firm	Bought by	Pharmaceutical Firm
Pharmaton (Switzerland)		Boehringer Ingelheim
Doktor Mann (Germany)		Bausch & Lomb
Klinge (Germany)		Fujisawa
Mack (Germany)		Pfizer
Plantorgan (Germany)		Sanofi
Asta Medica (Germany)		Degussa
Woelm Pharma (Germany)		Johnson & Johnson/Merck
Heumann (Germany)		Searle
Fink (Germany)		SmithKline Beecham
Dr. Much (Germany)		American Home Products
Quest (Canada)		Boehringer Ingelheim
Kali Chemie (Canada)		Solvay
Nattermann (Germany)		Rhone Poulenc Rohrer
Kanold (Germany)		Boehringer Ingelheim

Source: The European Phytomedicines Market--Figures, Trends, Analyses, by Jorg Grunwald, PhD; *HerbalGram* 34, Summer 1995

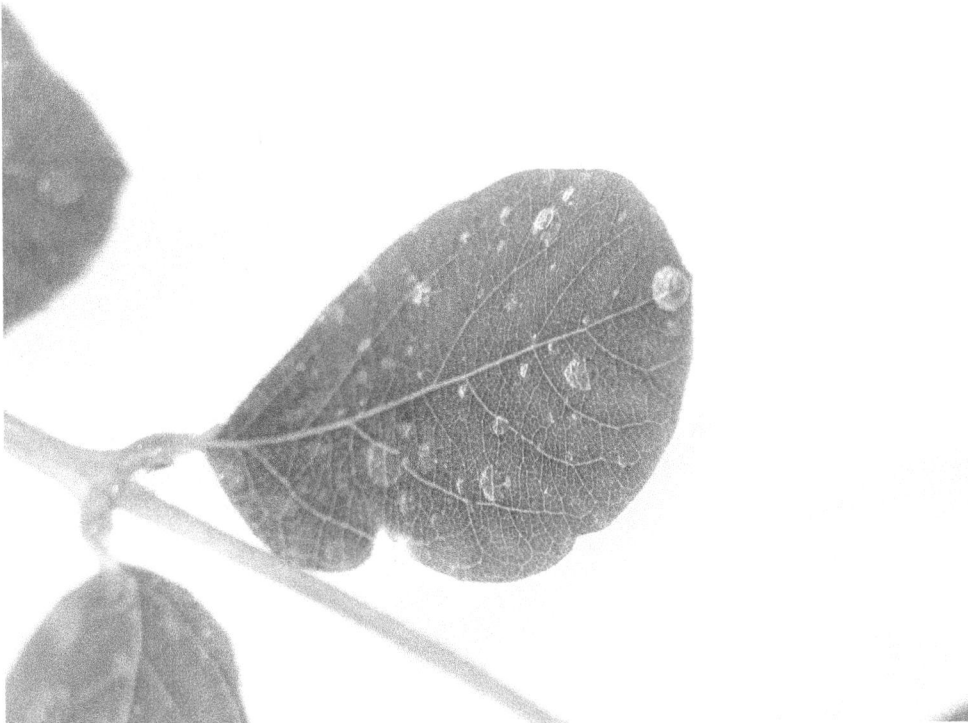

2006–

- **Florida lobbyists again** introduce a restrictive licensing bill that will prevent anyone other than graduates of CNME schools to practice if licensure is reinstated. H1261 and S2678 fail to restore licensure to the State of Florida.

2007–

- **The National Board of Naturopathic Medical Examiners** (NBNME) is established in Idaho, and administers a new examination, the United States Naturopathic Licensing Examination (USNLE). It is opposed by the Idaho chapter of the American Association of Naturopathic Physicians, but approved by the Idaho Association of Naturopathic Physicians*. **A fierce response to this is launched by the CNME, which insists that its NPLEX shall be the only accepted national board exam for the entire country.**

- **The International Society of Naturopathic Physicians** returns from dormancy. The organization had not been functioning for some years, but was revived by practitioners much like the ones who founded it back in 1938--moderates with medical training but not pseudo-medical in their philosophy. The ISNP would grant membership to all types of naturopaths without discrimination, and within a short time, there were deputy directors in Germany, France, England, Brazil, Cyprus, Puerto Rico, Poland, Hong Kong, Indonesia, and Japan. Its online journal *International Naturopath* became celebrated for its clinical orientation and, in the words of one reviewer, "refreshing lack of academic gobbledygook."

- **Washington State legislature is successfully lobbied to expand naturopathic scope** of practice to include **prescriptive rights, ability to give injections, perform minor surgery,** and greater in-office procedures.

- **Approximately 950 students were enrolled in the six CNME-accredited schools** (two in Canada) in 2007—a far cry from the small numbers when National and Bastyr were the only pseudo-medical schools. The population of pseudo-medical naturopaths begins to snowball.

- **Naturopathic Digest, an online journal, begins publication.** After some months of successful operation and having accumulated 7,700 subscribers, the executive editor apologized to his readers for including certain segments of the naturopathic population who were not qualified to receive their publication.

He stated, "Unfortunately, we were not completely aware of the significant educational chasm that exists between those who have graduated from CNME-accredited colleges and those who have not...we have come to recognize that providing information to providers who lack an essential scholarly foundation does little more than provide the appearance of credibility where it has not been earned. To the extent that this has been the case, we apologize to the profession."

Absolutely serious about this, the editor said that they intended to personally phone or e-mail anyone whose credentials they could not verify otherwise. "We are committed to restricting our circulation to only naturopathic doctors who are licensed and/or graduates of CNME-accredited colleges, as well as students from CNME-accredited programs and companies that support the naturopathic medical profession," he claimed.

Then the boast: "Compared to our January issue, we have eliminated 2,683 individuals who did not meet our requirements to receive the publication.⍰"

Over two thousand people were struck from the subscription rolls because they were not part of the community that considers itself to be made up of "real" naturopaths*.

---

* Minutes of the Idaho Board of Naturopathic Medical Examiners, Oct. 2007

- **National University of Health Sciences** (Lombard, Illinois) begins offering a pseudo-medical naturopathic program, the fifth in the U.S. It is the descendent of the school originally derived from the merger of Lindlahr's College of Naturopathy and National College of Chiropractic.

- **The Florida Senate Health Care Committee defeated 7-2 a bill to re-establish licensing** for naturopaths there. This was the third year in a row such a bill had been introduced. I.W. Lane College of Naturopathic Medicine, located in Winter Park, Florida, was instrumental in lobbying for licensure, and was supported by the AANP and told the school would have CNME candidacy status as an accredited school. However, when the bill reached committee, the CNME reversed itself and Lane's graduates would not have been eligible for licensure. Lad Santiago, DC, ND, pointed out to the Orlando Medical News* that I.W. Lane's proposed curriculum was more advanced and up to date than any of the CNME schools'. "Their intent was to create a monopoly so that naturopaths could only come from one particular set of schools," Santiago said. "They wanted to control the profession in the state of Florida."♦

- **Minnesota passes a law registering naturopaths.** It becomes the sixteenth state to allow only pseudo-medical naturopaths to practice. The law does not restrict applicants to have graduated from CNME-recognized schools, allowing graduates of "a degree granting college or university that prior to the existence of CNME, offered a full-time structured curriculum in basic sciences and supervised patient care, comprising a doctoral naturopathic medical education that is at least 132 weeks in duration". However, elsewhere the law states that in order to be registered, the

*"Future Practice of Naturopathic Medicine in Florida Uncertain" by Matthew Henry; *Orlando Medical News*, May 2008

♦ The president of Central States College confided to the author that the same thing happened when a licensing bill was considered in Ohio: CNME representatives were supportive of the school's accreditation until the bill was before committee; then they reversed their stance and disallowed Central States graduates to be licensed under the proposed law.

applicant must have passed the NPLEX examination —a test that only graduates of CNME schools are allowed to sit for. This is a "catch-22" that will preclude the possibility of any traditional or classical naturopaths practicing in that state.

> "As much as our curriculum taxes students with overabundant left-brain courses, NPLEX drives the nail into the coffin...The fact that these exams are comprised of multiple-choice questions should be enough to indicate the absurdity of using such an examination system to ensure that our doctors are prepared for practice. Perhaps they are prepared to practice like medical doctors, whose method of treatment revolves around formula-based treatments for specific diseases. Have not the students demonstrated their capacity to memorize for exams by having procured university degrees? All students demonstrate by passing the NPLEX exams is their capacity to memorize information. This doesn't indicate that they are ready for practice."
>
> --Daniel Block, ND
> *The Revolution of Naturopathic Medicine*,
> 2003 Collective Co-op Publishing, Page 97

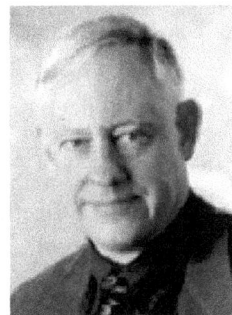

- **Bill Mitchell, ND dies.** Mitchell was a professor and one of the co-founders of Bastyr University. Renowned for his knowledge of botanical medicines, he was considered one of the last representatives of traditional Naturopathy within the realm of modern naturopathic medicine. While still respecting a science-based approach, he retained a love for Naturopathy's historical applications and vision. He more than once expressed dismay at the modern naturopath's rush to prescribe synthetic drugs, or treat in a this-for-that fashion. Mitchell's own inquisitiveness constantly led him to question just why a disease process was present, and fulfilled the naturopathic precept *Tolle Causum* (Look for the Cause).

- **Idaho repeals requirement of licensing of naturopathic physicians and dissolves the Board of Naturopathic Medical Examiners** as a result of several years of impasse between the pseudo-medical members on the board and traditional and classical naturopaths on the board.[*]

Senator Joyce Broadsword noted the "total disagreement" between the Idaho Chapter of the American Association of Naturopathic Physicians (pseudo-medical) and the Idaho Association of Naturopathic Physicians (traditional). The AANP chapter wanted licensees to have graduated only from a CNME school, and would be granted the right to perform minor surgery and have prescriptive privileges. The IANP wanted both traditional naturopaths and naturopathic physicians eligible for licenses.

As it stands, unlicensed naturopaths may still practice in Idaho, using heat, water, light, air, and massage as they have traditionally done. The AANP chapter says this "unfairly limits" their practices, because they cannot diagnose and write prescriptions, or perform surgical procedures.

Rather than allow both types of naturopaths to be licensed, the AANP contingent agreed to repeal licensure altogether.

Board of Naturopathic Medical Examiners member Brenda Grogan, ND, who supported the more liberal standard, summed it up:

"It's a political issue where somebody is scared to death they are going to lose their monopoly over Naturopathy. We've tried to talk it out. I don't care what you do, you could bend over backward and spin around 10 times, you're never going to get agreement, because there's two different philosophies."[♦]

Published in the *Idaho Statesman* on 02/24/09:

NATUROPATH LICENSING: Idaho needs a new law to protect against untrained doctors

The American Association of Naturopathic Physicians supports both the licensure of naturopathic physicians and the state Senate's vote to repeal the Idaho naturopathic licensing law ("Idaho Senate approves naturopath bill," Feb. 2). The licensing board has proven it is unable to generate rules that ensure that prescriptions are written by doctors who have trained in schools accredited through the U.S. Department of Education.

The AANP and our Idaho physicians, all of whom are licensed in other jurisdictions, stand firm in our commitment to patient safety. Any compromise that allows graduates of diploma mills (who have no clinical training to diagnose and treat chronic disease) to perform minor surgery and prescribe pharmaceuticals to unsuspecting citizens is unacceptable.

We encourage the Idaho House to take the Senate's lead, put an end to bad government and repeal this flawed law. Game over. We stand committed to Idaho residents and the passage of a good law, transparent regulations, and access to quality naturopathic medicine delivered by doctors who have trained at accredited schools, passed a nationally recognized exam and certify they are not felons.

Once again, the "accredited by the U.S. Department of Education" argument is being made.

---

[*] "Naturopath Repeal Clears Committee"; *The Spokesman-Review,* Jan. 27, 2009

[♦] "Naturopathic Licensing On The Rocks", by John Miller; *The Spokesman-Review* Jan. 22, 2009

- **The State of Oregon passes a bill broadening the scope of practice for NDs.** Their prescribing authority since the 1950s was limited to only natural substances, but now **synthetic drugs have been added to the naturopathic formulary.** Only pseudo-medical naturopaths may practice in Oregon.

- **A bill to broaden the scope of practice in Hawaii** was first vetoed by Governor Lingle but then was overridden, resulting in some **synthetic drugs, minor surgery, and parenteral (intravenous) therapy** being added to NDs' legal scope. Only pseudo-medical naturopaths may practice in Hawaii.

- **California's Bureau of Naturopathic Medicine is eliminated by Governor Schwarzenegger and placed as a committee under the Osteopathic Board.** Two NDs are added to the Osteopathic Board. The licensing law for pseudo-medical naturopaths was due to sunset in 2010, but this re-organization extends the law until 2013.

Discussing the California licensing law that also allows traditional NDs to practice and call themselves "naturopaths", naturopathic physician Stephen Sporn comments:

"…giving up the title 'naturopath' to the mail order group was not necessary in my opinion…Recent graduates don't have a sense of history and **their orientation tends towards trying to get along with everyone, and 'everyone has a right to do what they want'. This compromise saddens me.**" (emphasis ours)

(*Naturopathy Around The World,* by Hans Baer and Stephen Sporn, 2009 Nova Science Pub., p. 64)

Legal protectionism

- four states use and restrict the title "Doctor of Naturopathic Medicine"
- four states use and restrict the title "Naturopathic Doctor"
- four states use and restrict the title "Doctor of Naturopathy".
- seven states use and restrict the title "Naturopathic Physician".
- one state uses and restricts the title "Naturopath".

"It is my experience that in states that do not have licensure, in communities where you find a full-time traditional naturopath and a pseudo-medical naturopath, the traditional naturopath tends to have a bigger practice and a higher patient success rate. That ought to tell you something."

--Dr. Robert Thiel

The alliance of naturopathic schools under the mantle of the CNME's accreditation have opposed attempts at bridge programs where those with training elsewhere can complete their requirements for the ND degree at a CNME school.

But NCNM has a history of granting naturopathic degrees to other health care providers who did not graduate from exclusively naturopathic schools. This quote is from their 1975 catalogue:

> "The National College of Naturopathic Medicine's doctoral transfer post-graduate division was established by the college to meet the increasing demands of doctors licensed in other professions to obtain N.D. degrees and training. Realizing that the modern role of education is changing, and that licensed practitioners established in practice may not be able to quit practice to study Naturopathy, special arrangements were made with naturopathic associations recognized by other states and provincial licensing bodies, to teach clinical study leading to a Doctor of Naturopathy (N.D.) degree."

A perennially embarrassing situation for the now-dominant pseudo-medical naturopathic community is the sweeping of inconvenient facts under the carpet. One issue is that of ND degrees being issued by them under dubious circumstances in the past, which undermines their argument against traditional naturopaths boasting of "unearned degrees".

But the last sentence in the previous quote from the NCNM catalogue also illuminates another history revision on the part of the CNME: the commonly-held insistence that the ND granted to graduates of accredited schools stands for "Doctor of Naturopathic *Medicine*". As one can see from the above quote, the "Doctor of Naturopathy" degree was being granted even in the era of modern naturopathic medicine, and by the pseudo-medical schools. It was not until outright war broke out between the traditional naturopaths and the pseudo-medical naturopaths that the meaning of the degree was ever in question. With the burgeoning number of graduates of other programs such as Clayton and Trinity, the administration of the pseudo-medical

schools scrambled to differentiate their ND degree from that of the short course-type program. "They have studied Naturopathy," they seem to say, "but *we* are trained in naturopathic *medicine*."

While the distinction is not unreasonable, common sense would dictate that "ND" would not stand for "Doctor of Naturopathic Medicine". The uncommon NMD degree, awarded by at least two of the older (non-CNME-accredited) colleges*, was clearly delineated on those schools' diplomas as including the word "medicine". Yet for some reason, the CNME colleges have not chosen to grant this degree. Instead, peculiarly, they claim that their "ND" not only *really* means "Doctor of Naturopathic Medicine", but that it *always* did.

It may seem absurd that such a claim would go unchallenged by the current generation of naturopathic students, especially if they have access to historical documents at their schools. But few seem to have a quarrel over this and other issues because they are steeped in a deep hatred of traditional naturopaths, whom they believe to have stifled the profession while being a danger to the public. The CNME schools have fomented a fierce loathing in several generations of graduates, who are otherwise caring and benevolent practitioners.

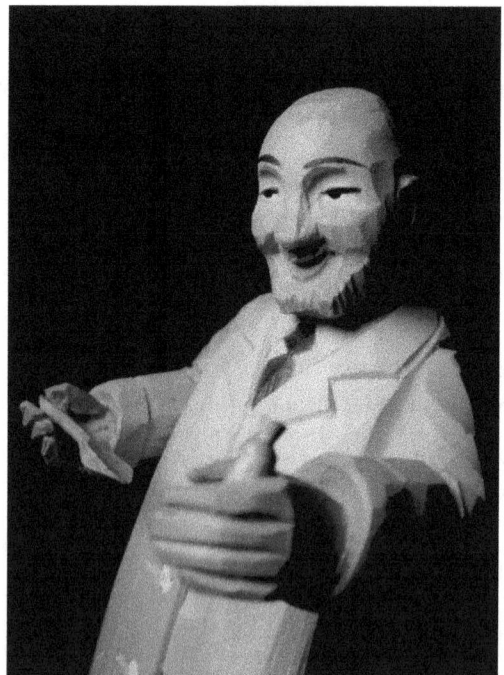

© Sarah Klockars-Clauser

* First National University and Central States College both historically granted this degree.

- **The District of Columbia Health Profession Licensing Administration was lobbied by the AANP to discontinue licenses for registered naturopaths**, while keeping intact the licenses for "naturopathic physicians". The two-tier licensing established in 2004 is abandoned with the 2010 expiration of several hundred traditional and classical naturopaths' registrations. The relatively few licenses issued to pseudo-medical naturopaths are renewed.

- **The International Society of Naturopathic Physicians web site is persistently and repeatedly hacked**, causing disruption in communication between the organization and its members all over the world. Viruses were periodically transmitted by email to the officers whose email addresses were listed. Two computers "crashed" as a result. Then attempts were made to compromise the private member section of the web site and to harvest the email addresses of all members. Finally, data was impregnated that linked the ISNP with a bank fraud operation in Ireland. International authorities alerted the ISNP to the attempt to implicate the organization, and the web site would eventually be taken down as a result. The ISNP, operating on a limited budget and composed of older members who were not fully part of the computer age, was not able to put out all the fires being lit around it.

The majority of the dozens of suspicious contacts with the web site emanated from IP addresses located in Kenmore, Washington and Mountain View, California. Even early on, there were disquieting signs that the ISNP was under scrutiny by hostile sources. ISNP President George Yuhasz noted that in the first 24 hours after uploading the web site, there were 273 views made, and the site would not yet appear on search engines for months. "Someone out there," he said, "knew what we were doing and didn't like it."

> Naturopaths practicing in unlicensed states have traditionally been able to point to the recognition by another state where they did hold licenses in order to prove their legitimacy—traditional naturopaths and pseudo-medical naturopaths alike. The District of Columbia is one district where they all maintained licenses.
>
> At the time of this writing, the District of Columbia has discontinued the licenses of 822 traditional and classical naturopaths, and granted licenses to only 22 pseudo-medical "naturopathic physicians", due to the lobbying efforts of the AANP and CNME.

> "Here is something curious. If you do an Internet search for Naturopathy on Euro countries' search engines, like England or Germany, the first link that comes up is Bastyr University. Now why would a school in Kenmore, Washington have to advertise in other countries? It is obvious that worldwide domination is their plan, not just an American monopoly."
>
> --Post on the ISNP member forum

- Bastyr University and Fred Hutchinson Cancer Research Center receive a **$3.1 million NIH grant for integrative breast cancer research.**

- **Bastyr receives a $4.52 million NIH grant** for the Bastyr/UW Oncomycology Translational Research Center to study the healing effects of Asian medicinal mushrooms on breast and prostate cancer.

- **Bastyr University announces its intention to establish a second campus** in California by 2012.

- **Clayton College of Natural Health, source of online courses for naturopaths and nutritionists, closes its virtual doors.** The institution most maligned by pseudo-medical naturopaths, its alumni were and are consistently criticized as "dangerous correspondence course graduates". While outnumbering graduates of CNME schools by several times, these "traditional naturopaths" find themselves increasingly unable to practice in the face of exclusionary licensing laws, despite the fact that they have been, as a group, very effective clinically with few instances of adverse events.

It is **incontestable** that naturopaths with less education, fewer tools, and no falling back on allopathic measures or synthetic drugs, consistently **cured people for the entire 20th Century.**

There exists no compelling argument that their modern-day counterparts should be barred from practice simply because one faction chooses to have a more medical education and presentation than the other.

To gain a proper perspective, one must realize that while the pseudo-medical naturopath wants to prevent the traditional naturopath from practicing, the orthodox medical doctor wants to prevent the pseudo-medical ND from practicing. While one fish is swallowing a smaller fish, a much larger fish is bearing down on him as well.

In 2006, The American Medical Association issued Resolution 209, specifically decrying the licensure of naturopaths and expressly opposing it.

They want to "...ensure that non-physician scope of practice is determined by training, experience, and demonstrated competence" (and of course even the pseudo-medical "accredited" naturopathic schools fall short of their standard). The AMA says clearly that it will "actively oppose legislation allowing non-physicians to engage in the practice of medicine."*

The biggest "fish" of all--the allopathic fish-- may make the disputes between the two naturopathic camps a moot point. If the medical orthodoxy is compelled to do so, it can probably eliminate all types of practitioners that it considers "non-physicians"--naturopaths, chiropractors, acupuncturists, etc. It has that kind of power. **What is likely, though, is that the modern ND will gradually be taken into the medical establishment as a second-class provider, as long as he or she is using the prescription pad and practicing "green allopathy".**

What we will probably never see again is the abundance of more traditional naturopaths, in the mold of Benedict Lust's generation.

> "Naturopathic physicians are the modern day science based primary care doctor."
>
> (From the AANP's Alliance Legislative Workbook, a guide for those lobbying legislators)

---

* American Medical Association House of Delegates, *License of Naturopaths,* Resolution 209 (A-06); Reports of the Board of Trustees, November 2006

Academic Snobbery

Graduates of CNME-accredited schools unhesitatingly repeat what they were told in school about those "correspondence school quacks" (like Clayton graduates). The promotional literature of these graduates typically mentions not only that he or she graduated from a "four year, accredited residential medical program" but also that there are "some people calling themselves naturopathic doctors who have only taken home-study courses." The message—sometimes implied, sometimes overt—is that the public should beware these dangerous pretenders.

A July 2003 report♦ released by the Department of Education, however, observes that 56% of the country's two- and four-year degree-granting institutions offer distance education courses.

Meanwhile, CNME-approved schools offer online degrees, the very thing that pseudo-medical naturopaths decry. The University of Bridgeport, for example, offers an online Master of Science in Clinical Nutrition. They state on their website: "The program provides this comprehensive study to individuals with busy schedules who would otherwise not be able to complete a graduate program without interrupting their work schedules."*

In fact, the number of video courses available to pseudo-medical naturopaths total over 200, and are an average length of only two hours. Such courses are available to students and graduates alike.

So one practitioner who simply offers dietary and nutritional advice with a degree from Clayton is a "dangerous" and "poorly-trained" healthcare provider, while a graduate of *Bridgeport's* distance program is a recognized and seemingly competent practitioner. This is the double standard being put forth to the public today.

There are over a hundred regionally accredited colleges and universities offering accredited courses in a non-resident mode. The Distance Education and Training Council (DETC) estimates that more than four million students participate in online courses. While "diploma mills" do exist, the overwhelming majority of distance-learning programs are nothing of the kind. Institutions of higher learning that have undergone independent review and have met the standards of regional accreditation clearly have no problem with nonresident degree programs. Harvard Medical School has online courses! Why, then, do the Council for Naturopathic Medical Education (CNME) and the American Association of Naturopathic Physicians (AANP) perpetuate the idea that any school that offers distance-learning courses is a "diploma mill"?

Any traditional or classical naturopath will say this: The AANP created the CNME and continues to dominate it. They want to insure that no schools except the ones they control (and profit from) can be accredited. As a result, all revenues for naturopathic education flow down one path.

This has the other intended effect of ultimately eliminating competition from naturopaths with a different vision. Simply put, it is making extinct an entire profession that has been accessible to those without much money. As requirements—and expenses—for naturopathic students continue to climb, the new naturopathic medical community mirrors the changes that took place years ago in the conventional medical field: Medical education became the province of the upper middle class and was beyond the means of the masses.

This explains the psychology of the pseudo-medical naturopath today, who righteously feels "Why should *they* be able to do what I do when I spent all that money and all those years?" It is easy to see why they are so vehement in their discrediting of other types of naturopaths.

♦ *Distance Education at Degree-Granting Institutions: 2000-2001*, National Center for Education Statistics (NCES) 2003
* http://www.bridgeport.edu/academics/graduate/nutrition

The American Association of Naturopathic Physicians proudly states* "Graduates of accredited naturopathic medical schools are required to have more hours of study in basic sciences and clinical sciences than graduates of Yale or Standford medical schools."

Yet, traditional naturopathic schools require more credit hours in *naturopathic* subjects than the CNME-accredited schools. Traditional naturopathic schools (such as First National, Trinity, Westbrook, Canyon, Clayton, etc.) have offered a greater selection of naturopathic courses as well. The pseudo-medical CNME schools concentrate on science courses, many of which are not germane to the practice of traditional Naturopathy but boost the students' confidence that they are at the pinnacle of the field.

It is interesting to note that, despite attempts to present a unified profession, the five U.S. pseudo-medical naturopathic schools do not all offer the same courses. Likewise, some practices that are typically listed as naturopathic modalities are not even taught at all schools. The number of hours required for strictly *naturopathic* courses at pseudo-medical schools do not meet the standards of Britain and Europe, yet the non-CNME schools (traditional schools) do meet those standards.

More disturbing is the question: Are the required "clinical practice hours" of the modern naturopathic physician sufficient training for the practice of the invasive medical procedures that their scope of practice increasingly includes? Remember, this training is not undergone in a hospital setting, so the usual comparison between them and medical doctors is something of a stretch. A recent online survey showed that 85% of naturopathic physicians polled are in favor of actively pursuing prescriptive rights in all states.✠

Anyone who stops and thinks will reason that no one can be expected to master *both* conventional medicine and natural medicine in the same length of time it formerly took for either one. Medical doctors feel that the new naturopaths have inadequate training in medicine. Traditional and classical naturopaths feel that they have inadequate training in Naturopathy. In the end, the modern ND may be something that is, as the old expression goes, neither fish nor fowl. But their numbers (now reaching 6,000), and their political might, continue to grow—just as their predecessors, the traditional and classical naturopaths, continue to dwindle.

*- *Naturopathic and Major Medical Schools: Comparative Curricula*; document from the AANP.
✠- www.ndolc.com/node/45